PSYCHOLOGY AND
ETHNOLOGY

Founded by C. K. Ogden

The International Library of Psychology

ANTHROPOLOGY AND PSYCHOLOGY
In 6 Volumes

PSYCHOLOGY AND ETHNOLOGY

W H R RIVERS

Edited with a Preface and Introduction
by G Elliot Smith

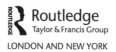

Routledge
Taylor & Francis Group

LONDON AND NEW YORK

First published in 1926 by
Routledge, Trench, Trubner & Co., Ltd.

Reprinted in 1999 by
Routledge
2 Park Square, Milton Park, Abingdon, Oxon, OX14 4RN

Simultaneously published in the USA and Canada by Routledge

711 Third Avenue, New York, NY 10017

Transferred to Digital Printing 2007

Routledge is an imprint of the Taylor & Francis Group, an informa business

First issued in paperback 2013

© 1926 W H R Rivers

British Library Cataloguing in Publication Data
A CIP catalogue record for this book
is available from the British Library

Psychology and Ethnology

ISBN 978-0-415-20954-0 (hbk)
ISBN 978-0-415-86434-3 (pbk)

CONTENTS

PREFACE

THIS volume of essays is issued in fulfilment of a promise made to Dr Rivers to collect and publish in book form a series of his memoirs on ethnological subjects that are scattered in volumes not readily accessible to students. In particular he was anxious that the articles on "The Disappearance of Useful Arts," published at Helsingfors in the *Festskrift Tillägnad Edvard Westermarck* (1912), and "The Contact of Peoples" from the *Essays presented to William Ridgeway* (1913) should be more widely known. Professor Westermarck and Sir William Ridgeway gave their ready consent to the reprinting of these two essays and thus made possible the preparation of this volume. Dr Robert H. Lowie kindly permitted the republication of "Sun-Cult and Megaliths in Oceania" that originally appeared in the *American Anthropologist*, of which he is the Editor. The Syndics of the Cambridge University Press have authorized the reprinting of "Freud's Concept of the 'Censorship'," which is an Appendix of Dr Rivers's *Instinct and the Unconscious*.

The difficult task of selecting from the various published essays and addresses and the hitherto unpublished manuscripts the series for inclusion in this volume has been made easier by Mr W. J. Perry's advice. In addition he has collected the bibliographical references for several chapters of the book, in particular that dealing with "Irrigation and the Cultivation of Taro." This important memoir was communicated to the Manchester Literary and Philosophical Society in 1916 (see *Nature*, 1916, p. 214) : but Dr Rivers refrained from publishing it until he had collected more evidence. He had almost (but not quite) completed this work at the time of his death. The map (p. 263) prepared by Mr C. Daryll Forde of University College shows only the sites actually mentioned by Dr Rivers and is not a complete chart of the distribution of Taro cultivation.

The essays collected in this volume form a very heterogeneous collection. Some of them are very slight, in fact little more than notes on subjects that Dr Rivers intended to investigate further. But, diverse as they are, they all have this in common : their essential theme is the search for the psychological motives that impelled men to develop customs and beliefs in particular ways. For Dr Rivers, who was a psychologist first and an ethnologist afterwards, every problem in ethnology was essentially psychological.

Mr H. J. Massingham kindly undertook the difficult task of preparing the manuscript for printing, the grouping of the chapters and the index.

G. E. S.

INTRODUCTION

DR RIVERS AND THE NEW VISION IN ETHNOLOGY

To appreciate the full significance of the services rendered by Dr Rivers to Ethnology, it is essential to consider his scientific training and the circumstances that drew him into ethnological research and shaped his aims.

As a fieldworker, he was conspicuously successful in collecting exact and reliable information. This was due largely to the sympathetic understanding of the people of lowly culture whom he was studying and the strict scientific discipline that eliminated bias and gave free scope for his insight in interpreting the information he collected. The mere collection and tabulation of facts, however, were not his real interests, but merely the essential preparation for the investigation of the psychological problems that lie at the heart of Ethnology. The interpretation of social practices, beliefs and customs, appealed to him chiefly as a means of approach to the mental processes that were involved. The thoughts and behaviour of any community were worthy of study as a means of understanding the psychology of mankind as a whole.

A quarter of a century ago, when Ethnology had acquired a strong hold on his interests, the problem of the social functions of the mother's brother loomed large in his programme of work. In attempting to appreciate the circumstances in Rivers's own case that led to his adoption of Anthropology as the main interest in his life, it is curious to note the efforts of his maternal uncle, Dr James Hunt, to focus Rivers's interest in anthropological work from his earliest youth. The year before Rivers was born, Dr Hunt founded and became the first president of the Anthropological Society. The Society began its work with the publication of an English translation of the book *Anthropologie der Naturvölker* by Dr Theodor Waitz, in which more attention was paid to the psychological aspects of Ethnology than had previously been done in any work on the subject. When Rivers was three weeks old, his uncle presented to him a copy of this translation, duly inscribed and signed, which is now before me as I write. In turning over the pages of this book, in which its owner took no interest whatever until thirty-five years after it was given to him, it is not a little curious to read the summary of the conclusions to which Waitz was led :—"Civilization is dependent more on historical events than on original mental endowment"—a point of view that Rivers himself adopted in the closing years of his life, when by a curious irony of fate Waitz had come to be regarded as one of the chief protagonists of a view that is almost the antithesis of this statement.

But Ethnology had no attractions for Rivers until his work in Psychology was responsible for drawing him into this field of investigation. When Dr Haddon in 1898 was framing the programme of work to be undertaken by the Cambridge Anthropological Expedition to the Torres Strait, he decided to make a serious attempt to investigate the psychology of the people. With this object in view, he persuaded Dr Rivers to organize and carry out the first systematic fieldwork in the experimental psychology of primitive people.

This interesting innovation, however, did more than bring practical Psychology into close co-ordination with Ethnology. For Rivers himself it opened up a new interest, and incidentally became a turning point in the history of Anthropology, as the Chapter on the *Ethnological Analysis of Culture* in this book indicates. Before 1898, Rivers was so little interested in Anthropology that he declined the valuable anthropological library collected by his uncle on the ground that such books were of no use to him. But eventually he was led into anthropology along the pathway of neurology and psychology. While his natural aptitude for such work should be freely admitted, it was largely due to chance that Rivers's interest became centred upon neurology. The position of House-Physician at St Bartholomew's Hospital had been offered to Dr E. G. Browne: but, in 1887, several months before he was due to take up this position, he went out to Persia and decided to devote himself to Oriental Studies, in which, later on, as lecturer in Persian, and afterwards as the Lord Almoner's Professor of Arabic at the University of Cambridge, he achieved high distinction. The vacancy thus created was filled by Rivers, who also was destined to attain in the University of Cambridge a unique position in another branch of the Humanities, as well as in Science.

In 1888, Rivers thus became a House-Physician at St Bartholomew's Hospital under Dr Gee, whose interest in neurology determined the kind of work

Rivers had to do. When he was only twenty-four years of age, Rivers wrote a report on " A Case of Spasm of the Muscles of the Neck causing Protrusion of the Head," and a year later a communication on " Delirium and its Allied Conditions " (St. Bartholomew's Hospital Reports, Vols. XXIV and XXV). These leanings towards neurology and psychiatry led him to the National Hospital for the Paralysed and Epileptic in Queen Square, where he became a House-Physician in 1891. There he came under the influence of Hughlings Jackson and assisted Victor Horsley in his pioneer operations on the brain, which opened a wonderful vista of possibilities for a young psychologist. But a factor that was even more potent than the stimulating influence of Victor Horsley, or even contact with the mastermind of the great neurological philosopher, Hughlings Jackson, was the association at Queen Square with Dr Henry Head, who had just returned from Germany full of enthusiasm for Hering and his work on vision. Under such circumstances, Rivers's interest became more definitely fixed on the borderline between neurology and psychology. He was working at the problems of hysteria and neurasthenia, the analogies between delirium and mania, and soon felt the urgent need for the closer cooperation between neurology and psychology. In 1892 he studied at Jena, where he recorded in his diary that on his return home he would devote himself to the investigation of insanity and work as much as possible at psychology.

Hence, on his return to England in 1892, he began work at the Bethlem Royal Hospital. In the following year, he lectured at Guy's Hospital on the more strictly psychological aspects of mental disease and at University College, London, on experimental psychology. In the same year, at Sir Michael Foster's invitation, he began teaching the physiology of the sense organs in Cambridge, and returned to Germany for a short period of study under Professor Kräpelin at Heidelberg, more especially with reference to the effects of drugs on bodily and mental fatigue.

His pupil, Dr Charles Myers, from whose account (W. H. R. Rivers, *Psychology and Politics*, Kegan Paul, 1923) of Rivers's career in psychology I have freely drawn in the preceding paragraphs, speaks from personal knowledge when he says, " At Cambridge Rivers set himself to plan one of the earliest systematic practical courses in experimental psychology in the world, certainly the first in this country. In 1897 he was officially recognized by the University, being elected to the newly - established lectureship in Physiological and Experimental Psychology." Three years later, the masterly treatise on vision in Schäfer's *Physiology* set the seal on his reputation as the chief authority on this branch of physiology. Hence, when in the following year he embarked upon his first anthropological expedition, Rivers devoted himself especially to the investigation of vision in the Torres Strait Islanders.

The problems raised by his first experience of field-work stimulated him to examine other peoples. In the winter of 1900-1901, he went out to Egypt and at the archæological camp of Dr Randall-MacIver and the late Mr Anthony Wilkin at El Amrah near Abydos in Upper Egypt, he investigated the colour vision of the workmen engaged in their investigations. Incidentally and quite unwittingly, Dr Rivers was responsible for drawing me into anthropology. At his suggestion I visited El Amrah to study what until then was the unknown phenomenon of the natural preservation of the brain in the crania of predynastic Egyptians. So many other problems in anatomy presented themselves for solution that before long I had become definitely committed to the study of the anthropology of Egypt. In the following year, Dr Rivers went out to India to embark upon his first independent research in pure ethnology—the study of the Todas.

According to Dr Myers, his psychological investigations among the Torres Strait Islanders, Egyptians and Todas will ever stand as models of precise, methodical observations in the field of ethnological psychology. Nowhere does he disclose more clearly the admirably scientific bent of his mind—his insistence on scientific procedure, his delight in scientific analysis, and his facility in adapting scientific methods to novel experimental conditions. He reached the conclusion that no substantial difference exists between the visual acuity of civilized and uncivilized peoples, but that the latter show a very definite diminution in sensibility to blue.

When Dr Rivers embarked upon his first independent expedition, he worked both at psychology and at the investigation of religion and sociology. But the two lines of work were kept more or less distinct the one from the other. The psychological research was essentially physiological in nature (*British Journal of Psychology*, 1905, p. 321) and had no close or direct bearing on the other branch of his study, the results of which were published in the volume entitled *The Todas* (1906). In the Preface to the latter he explains— and the point is distinctive of Rivers's contribution to Ethnology—that in writing the book his object had been to make it, not merely a record of the customs and beliefs of a people, but also a demonstration of anthropological method. For, he continues, the great need of anthropology is for a more exact method, not only in collecting material, but also in recording it, so that readers may be able to assign its proper value to each fact, and may be provided with definite evidence which will enable them to estimate the probable veraciousness and thoroughness of the record.

Perhaps it was as a result of keeping his psychological and ethnological researches more or less distinct the one from the other that Rivers in 1906 did not appreciate the incompatibility of the views which four years later he was destined to repudiate. Thus in *The Todas* (p. 4) he states: "Perhaps the most definite result which modern research in Anthropology has brought out is the extraordinary similarity of custom throughout the world." "Customs apparently identical are found in races so widely separated geographically and so diverse ethnologically that it seems certain the customs must have developed in total independence of one another." But even at that time, when Rivers did not consciously dissent from the fashionable formula, one can detect the first step in the logical process that eventually led him to repudiate the doctrine of so-called psychic unity. Thus he states: "There seems to be an identity of idea actuating custom in peoples very different from one another in their surroundings and conditions of life." But it is an essential part of the doctrine associated with the names of Bastian and Tylor that similar customs and institutions come into existence and develop on the same lines *when the conditions are similar*.

It was not, however, until he had returned from another expedition—this time to Melanesia—and was engaged in the task of interpreting his results that the fact was brought home to him of their incompatibility with the currently accepted theory. In the Preface to *The History of Melanesian Society* (1914) he tells what happened with characteristic candour: "When *The Todas* was written, I had fully realized the insufficiency of current methods of collecting the facts of ethnography, but I was then under the sway of the crude evolutionary doctrine of the time, and did not see that the need for sound method was equally great in the theoretical treatment of these facts. It was only in the act of writing this book [*Melanesian Society*] that I came gradually to realize the unsatisfactory character of current ethnological methods. From that time, method again became my chief interest."

The history of this change of attitude is discussed more fully in the address on "The Ethnological Analysis of Culture" (1911), which is reprinted in this book. Although this change of view involved the admission of the reality of cultural diffusion, the attention of Dr Rivers became focussed upon the effects of the admixture of different cultures and their mutual influence one upon the other rather than upon the essential problems of diffusion itself. The essay on The Contact of Peoples in this volume deals with this phase of attitude, which is also developed more fully in the book *Medicine, Magic and Religion* (1924). But at the time (1915) the lectures included in the latter book were being written, Dr. Rivers was beginning to realize that he had pushed the theory of mixture of cultures further than the evidence warranted. In other words, he found that he was attempting to explain as the result of the blending of two elements in Melanesia practices that were introduced into the region from elsewhere in essentially the same complex form. As the facts relating to circumcision and incision were mainly responsible for convincing Dr Rivers that the hypotheses tentatively put forward in *The History of Melanesian Society* needed modification, the essay entitled "Circumcision, Incision and Sub-incision" has been included in this volume. At first sight there may not seem to be any justification for regarding such a topic as appropriate for inclusion in a book dealing with psychological problems. But it is the magico-religious purpose and the question of why these things were done that appealed to Dr Rivers. Hence the essay on "Circumcision," like those on "Massage in Melanesia" and "Sexual Relations and Marriage in Eddystone Island," and several other apparently irrelevant essays and notes, are really studies in the psychology of motives.

After completing *The History of Melanesian Society*, Dr Rivers visited Australia and New Zealand in 1914 and delivered the addresses on "The Problem of Australian Culture" and "The Peopling of Polynesia" that are printed for the first time in this volume. He revisited Melanesia before returning to England.

In the summer of 1915 he joined the Staff of the Military Hospital at Maghull where soldiers suffering from the mental effects of the stress and strain of trench warfare were being treated. Rivers threw himself into this work with intense enthusiasm. It appealed to him not only because it was interesting psychologically and of great practical importance as the means of dealing effectively with a national problem of rapidly increasing importance: but more particularly because he found that the measures taken to discover the causes of the soldiers' mental disabilities

b

were so similar to those he had been using in Melanesia to probe into the social and magico-religious problems of peoples of lowly culture.

During the arduous time Rivers spent in various Military Hospitals during the Great War, he often found relief in ethnological study. The essay on "Irrigation and the Cultivation of Taro" is one of the results of such diversions. But a far more important phenomenon of this double discipline was the effect upon his own outlook.

For he now began to integrate the processes of psychology and ethnology into one discipline.

The important books that were written during this period, *Instinct and the Unconscious*, *Conflict and Dream*, *Psychology and Politics*, *Medicine, Magic and Religion*, and *Social Organization* reveal the fact that for Rivers the barrier between his psychological and ethnological studies had been broken down and the two had become intimately blended the one with the other. The present series of essays affords a further testimony to the completeness of this fusion.

The effects of these events upon the interpretation of human thought and behaviour are far-reaching and of exceptional importance. In attempting to interpret their significance, I shall rely mainly upon Rivers's own statements.

In his Presidential Address to the Folk-Lore Society in 1922, he explained his views upon the relationship of psychology to ethnology. Although he was primarily considering folk-lore, it is clear from the context that his remarks apply with equal, or even greater, force to ethnology as a whole. Hence, I shall freely use the report of that address to express in his own words the conviction that the essential aim of every enquiry into the nature of custom and belief is to discover the psychological reasons in explanation of men's actions and thoughts.

Ethnology consists of something more than the collection of curiosities. The time has gone by when we can expect people to collect folk-lore, or any other kind of ethnological data, on account of its quaintness or its picturesqueness. It is necessary to provide a more definite motive and to show how it may contribute to our better understanding of man and his culture and to the solution of problems with which the student of human society is now confronted.

These problems are very diversified, but two important groups can be clearly distinguished, both having in common the fact that their solution seems most likely to be attained by the comparative study of belief and custom. The main interest of one of the two groups is historical. The problems it presents are attacked in the hope that through comparative study we may gain material by means of which to construct a history of human progress ; not a history dealing merely with the conflicts of civilized peoples, with the rivalries of kings and the battles of nations, but a history of the movements of thought ; of the long struggle of Man with his environment ; and of the countless institutions, beliefs and customs which have been the outcome of this struggle.

The other main group of problems which should provide an adequate motive for ethnology gains its interest from the fact that the comparative study of human custom and belief provides material for the psychologist. In the last resort, every custom and institution of human society is the outcome of mental activity. The history of institutions that has just been put forward as providing a motive for our interest has itself been determined in the main by mental factors. Its course has been dependent, partly on the nature of the psychological motives which have come into action during Man's struggle with his environment, both material and social, and partly on the psychological processes by which mental trends once adapted to crude and simple modes of life have been modified and developed to enable both the individual and the group to cope with the increasing complexity of human society.[1]

As he explains in the first essay in this book, the relation between psychology and the study of human culture is highly complex. On the one hand, the historian, the ethnologist and the folk-lorist look to the psychologist for knowledge of the motives and processes which have prompted and guided human progress. On the other hand, social interactions and the products of these interactions provide material for the psychologist. The modern psychologist is not content to study by means of introspection the modes of activity of his own mind. He supplements these, or even wholly substitutes for them, the observation of behaviour of the animal, of the child, of his fellow-men, especially under peculiar conditions and pre-eminently when they are the victims of disease, and last, but far from least, of the collective behaviour which has found expression in the political institutions, the economic processes, the religious rites, and the material and æsthetic arts of the different forms of human society.

At present the student of human custom and belief

[1] W. H. R. Rivers, *Instinct and the Unconscious*, 2nd ed., Cambridge, 1922 : *Conflict and Dream*, London, 1923.

can render a greater service to the psychologist than he can expect from him. The student of mind in the past, depending chiefly or wholly on introspection, has naturally had the individual as the main object of his interest and of his study. Valuable, indeed essential, as is the knowledge of the individual mind, it is clear that new factors must come into action in determining collective behaviour. We cannot be content to apply the findings of the psychology of the individual when we seek out the springs of social conduct. Social psychology needs material derived directly from the study of social behaviour, and for this material it must look to the observer of the rites, customs and institutions which are the objects studied by the ethnologist and the folk-lorist. In his Presidential Address to the Folk-Lore Society in 1921, he dealt with a problem in the study of which psychology can help the ethnologist. But the comparative study of rite and custom can help the psychologist in the solution of certain problems which are now an especial object of his interest. In dealing with the subject of symbolism Ethnology can render a clear guidance to psychology.

Many different lines of research are now leading students towards the conviction that symbolism is, and still more has been in the past, a process of vast importance in the history of human thought. Even to-day it is difficult to overestimate the importance of symbols in the behaviour of mankind. Especially important are they in collective behaviour, bringing into activity early phases of thought and sentiment which might seem to have passed into the background of the mental activity of the individual, at any rate of the more educated individual of the time. We have only to consider the importance among ourselves of the flag as a symbol of nationality and of the crown as a symbol of empire to see how great a hold symbolism still has upon the most advanced civilizations of the day. In many lines of study we are coming to see that such symbols as the flag and the crown are only conspicuous instances of the activity of a process which takes, and has taken, a leading part in the welfare of mankind in all places and at all times.

Strangely enough the special interest which modern psychology has come to take in symbolism is not due in the first place to the study of such cruder forms of human thought as are exemplified by the savage or the child, but has arisen out of the study of disease and of the dream. Students of those nervous and mental disorders which we call the psychoses and psycho-neuroses have come to see that many of the manifestations or symptoms of these disorders have a symbolic nature and are symbols of some underlying trouble which cannot come to consciousness in its true guise. The psycho-neurosis may be regarded as a symbolic expression of a deeply-seated trouble providing a solution of some situation with which the sufferer is unable to cope in its naked reality.

Again, the fantastic and irrational structure of the dream is regarded as a symbolic expression of some deeply-seated desire or anxiety which is not allowed to come to overt consciousness during the waking hours, and even when the control of the waking life has been removed in sleep finds expression only in symbolic form.

Those who have been led by their studies to the recognition of the great importance of symbolism in disease and dream have not stopped at that point. There is now an extensive literature in which attempts are made to bring the symbolism of myth and ritual into relation with modern views concerning its rôle in the dream and in disease. One of the most striking conclusions to which this comparative study has led some writers is that there is a universal system of symbolization among mankind ; that among all races of mankind and in the members of every race there is a tendency to symbolize certain thoughts by means of the same symbols, or at least by symbols having a close similarity to one another. This belief in a universal system of symbolization has been reached in the first place by the similarity which is found to exist in the nature of the symbols utilized by the morbid thought-processes of psychoneurosis and by such consciousness as remains active in sleep. Many attempts have been made to show that this universality of symbolism, which is believed to hold good of pathological or quasi-pathological processes, also applies to the myths and rites of the many peoples of the earth. This view needs to be critically examined. It will be necessary to consider certain problems with which we are confronted whenever the question of the universality of any manifestation of the human mind is being discussed. If it could·be shown that any human thought, such as the symbolization of good by the right hand and evil by the left, were universal, we should then have to decide whether this universality depends on an innate capacity for symbolization of this kind or whether it is the result of a common tradition so prevalent that it influences every member of the community and becomes, perhaps at an early stage of his life, part of the furniture of his mind. We have to decide whether the universal use of the symbol is due to heredity or to what Graham Wallas has fitly called "social heritage." [1] The advocates of the universality of symbolism, such as Jung and Freud and their disciples, seem to believe in the former alternative. The primordial thought-images of Jung which make up his collective unconscious are assumed to be hereditary, though it is difficult to find any clear expression of Jung's opinion on this point.

It is evident that the question whether certain systems of symbolization are or are not of universal distribution is closely related to the problem of the influence of the relative shares taken in the production of mental events by heredity and social heritage. If we find that certain symbols are really universal, there would be at least a *prima facie* case for the influence of heredity. If, on the other hand, no such universality is found, we shall have to look to social heritage for our explanation of the prevalence of the same mode of symbolism among different peoples or among the different members of one people.

Closely connected with this problem is another, which is now prominent in the thoughts of students of human custom, concerning the part taken by diffusion. If we should succeed in finding the universal distribution of a symbol, there would remain the further question whether it was universal because through heredity it had become part of the inherent equipment of the human mind, or whether the use of the symbol has been carried about the world by the movements of some body or bodies of men in whose system of thought the symbol was prominent. As has been

[1] *Our Social Heritage*, London, 1921.

pointed out by those who hold the former view, if it were found that the use of a symbol is indeed universal, the question whether it has been diffused or not is of no great importance, for we could hardly expect the use of a symbol to receive universal acceptation unless there was some disposition universally present in the human mind which made the use of the symbol fitting and natural. If, however, we find that the use of a symbol is not universal, and still more if we find that the peoples who use it show other clear evidence of influence from without, the fact of diffusion becomes of great significance, and the probability greatly in favour of the view that, wherever it is found, it is part of the social heritage.

In the address from which these statements are quoted, Dr Rivers makes a critical examination of the claims that have been made by followers of Freud to explain the similarities of myth and folk-lore, custom and belief, as different expressions of the so-called universal symbolism. To test these hypotheses he choses for consideration the subject of rebirth, with which so much of the Freudian contribution to ethnology is concerned. He brushes aside what he calls the fantastic speculation of assuming that even before birth a child has such almost superhuman prescience and acute powers of observation as to appreciate the association between the amniotic fluid and the act of birth. Then he proceeds to deal with the less frivolous aspects of the problem. After examining the geographical distribution and cultural associations of the symbolism of rebirth in religious ritual, Dr Rivers shows that it is not universal. By destroying the foundations of these assumptions of belief in typical symbols that were said to be innate in the minds of all mankind, Dr Rivers

has not only dealt a fatal blow to the Freudian interpretation of Ethnology, but also to Bastian's conception of *Elementargedanke*, of which the former is a
rationalization.

The modern doctrines of Ethnology—the supposition
that culture grew up independently and in much the
same way in widely separated areas—only received wide
acceptance when in 1871 Mr (later Sir) Edward Tylor
adopted it in his *Primitive Culture*. He acknowledged
his debt to Theodor Waitz and Adolf Bastian for the
idea; but the factor that played the chief part in
perverting him from the essentially diffusionist interpretation adopted in his earlier book (*The Early History
of Mankind*, 1865) was the conviction of the universality
of what he called animism. When Dr Rivers demonstrated that symbolism was not universal, he completely
undermined not only the Freudian interpretation of
ethnological data, but equally also that of Bastian and
Tylor.

In the essay called "The Ethnological Analysis of
Culture," which is reprinted here from his Presidential
Address to the Section of Anthropology at the British
Association in 1911, Dr Rivers explains how he was
forced to renounce a belief in Bastian's *Elementargedanke* and the idea of independent evolution based
on a community of thought. The essay on "Freud's
Concept of the 'Censorship'" has been included in this
volume to show that, while dissenting from the view
associated with the Freudian speculations in Ethnology,
Dr Rivers gave a qualified assent to the main principles
of psychological analysis.

The address on the *Ethnological Analysis of Culture*
marked an epoch not only in Dr Rivers's own career,
but also in the history of ethnology. He had been

working at the subject for more than twelve years without seriously questioning the validity of the hypothesis of the independent development of culture.

But when in 1910 he began to examine the evidence he had collected in Melanesia, the conclusion was brought home to him that his data could not be forced into harmony with the doctrine then fashionable in ethnology. To quote his own words: "I was led by my facts to see how much, in the past, I had myself ignored considerations arising from racial mixture and the blending of cultures"

The conviction was forced upon Dr Rivers in 1911 that if considerations of diffusion were eliminated from the comparative study of customs and beliefs the result was confusion. The modern hypothesis of the independent development of culture which Sir Edward Tylor adopted from Adolf Bastian subsequently became known as "evolution." The irony involved in the misuse of this irrelevant label cannot be fully appreciated unless the reader is reminded of the fact that Adolf Bastian was the friend and collaborator of Virchow in his reckless opposition to the whole conception of biological evolution. In the address called in the English version *Freedom in Science and Teaching* (1879), Haeckel refers to Bastian as the "enfant terrible" of the school (of opponents of evolution), who has been "well-nicknamed Acting Privy Counsellor of the Board of Confusion." The choice in ethnology is between accepting diffusion or the confusion of Bastian. Dr Rivers announced his decision in 1911.

But if this is the most signal service rendered by Dr Rivers it by no means represents the whole of the debt Ethnology owes him. He gave the subject scientific discipline, breadth of outlook and coherence with humanitarian studies. He established the intimate co-operation of Ethnology with Psychology —not the spurious psychology of Bastian's *Elementargedanke* or Freud's typical symbols, but the serious study of mental phenomena by methods conforming to scientific principles. The ultimate influence of Rivers's life-work will unquestionably be to bring anthropology back into conformity with the principle so lucidly expounded by Sir Edward Tylor when he wrote: "The notion of the continuity of civilization is no barren philosophic principle, but is at once made practical by the consideration that they who wish to understand their own lives ought to know the stages through which their opinions and habits have become what they are." "It is only when men fail to see the line of connexion in events, that they are prone to fall back upon the notions of arbitrary impulses, causeless freaks, chance and nonsense, and indefinite unaccountability."

These sane principles are none the less impressive because they appear, incongruously enough, in a book (*Primitive Culture*, 1871, p. 17) that inaugurated the wholesale process of defying them, which has now been happening for more than half a century. "To ingenious attempts at explaining by the light of reason things that want the light of history to show their meaning, much of the learned nonsense of the world has indeed been due." (*Op. cit.*, p. 18).

By relighting the lamp of history and reinforcing its illumination by the light of true reason, Dr Rivers had prepared the way for the elimination of much of the darkness and the learned nonsense from Ethnology.

G. ELLIOT SMITH.

PART I

PSYCHOLOGY

I

SOCIOLOGY AND PSYCHOLOGY [1]

IN a paper [2] read before the Sociological Society in 1913, and in some lectures [3] delivered at the London School of Economics in the same year, I put forward a view concerning the relation between Sociology and Psychology which it is the purpose of this chapter to consider more fully.

I must begin by stating briefly what I understand by psychology and sociology. I am sorry to have to spend time on a topic on which, it might be thought, there is general agreement, but a private criticism of my earlier work by one whose opinion I value highly has convinced me that this course is necessary. My critic wrote that he did not know in what sense I used the terms in question, and then proceeded to give definitions of his own which, if I had accepted them, would have reduced my whole position to an absurdity.

I use the term " psychology " for the science which deals with mental phenomena, conscious and unconscious. I am fully aware that, from the point of view of the psychologist, I am, begging the whole question as it interests him by my use of the word " mental." But, from the point of view of the student of society, the exact meaning of the word " mental " is of no great importance. The important matter to him is that whatever may be the exact meaning of the word " mental " adopted by psychologists, there is no danger

[1] From the *Sociological Review*, Autumn, 1916.
[2] " Survival in Sociology," *Sociological Review*, 1913, vol. vi, p. 293.
[3] *Kinship and Social Organization*, London, 1914.

of confusing mental processes with the social processes which
I regard as the subject-matter of sociology. The definition
of psychology I wish to exclude as a wholly inadequate one
of the relation between sociology and psychology is that of
McDougall [1]—that psychology is the science of the behaviour
of living things. This definition is so wide that it would
not only include the whole of sociology as ordinarily understood, but also economics, politics, and ethics. The definition
is so wide as to be useless if those subjects are to be distinguished as separate disciplines.

On passing to the meaning I attach to the term
" sociology," the first point to notice is that, just as it is
possible to describe any of our daily actions as individuals
without any reference .to the motives which prompt these
actions, so is it possible to describe the actions of human
beings as members of society without reference to motives.
In the case of individual actions, there is no need for their
co-ordinated study in such a manner as to make up a science ;
it is only when human actions are carried out in conjunction
with others, or involve the social welfare of others, that
we are entitled to speak of them as social actions. These
social actions as a whole form a body of organized processes
which can be described and classified, and their relations in
space and time studied. It is this description and classification, together with the study of these relations, which I regard
as the special subject-matter of sociology.

And, I may remark that, even so limited, sociology still
remains no small discipline. It would be possible, for instance, to write volumes on that group of social processes
which we sum up under the term " marriage," without the
use of a single psychological term referring to instincts,
emotions, sentiments, ideas or beliefs, without mentioning
such states as love, jealousy, and constancy, which everybody

[1] *Psychology, The Study of Behaviour*, London, 1912.

knows to stand in so close a relation to the social processes in question. It would probably be objected that by such treatment the subject had been deprived of all life.[1] While fully acknowledging that no treatment of marriage would be complete in which such topics as love and jealousy were ignored, such treatment is capable of producing valuable contributions to our knowledge. It would be a study in what might be called pure sociology.

It will, I trust, have become evident that the distinction I seek to make between sociology and social psychology is essentially one of method. We are now only at the threshold of the scientific study of human society. We are able to look back at a large amount of pioneer work by means of which facts have been garnered. It is now our task to establish methods and principles by means of which these facts may be used to build up one of those systematized and coherent bodies of knowledge which we call science. How little has been done towards the construction of such an edifice is shown by the widely divergent directions, of the attempts which have been made to this end and by the absence of generally accepted principles comparable with those upon which other sciences are based. This absence is so conspicuous that it has been possible, not merely to deny the existence of a science of sociology, but even to deny its possibility.[2]

To me, as to most students of the subject, the final aim of the study of society is the explanation of social behaviour in terms of psychology. The point upon which I wish to insist is one of method. We have to discover by what methods this aim may be attained. The solution of the problem which I propose is that the end at which we are aiming will be reached by proceeding along two paths, which, taking a parallel course

[1] Cf. R. R. Marett, *Folk-Lore*, xxv (1914), 21.
[2] Cf. H. G. Wells, *Sociological Papers*, London, 1907, vol. iii, p. 357.

at first, will gradually converge as they approach the goal. Those who follow one path will devote themselves to the study of the body of customs and institutions which make up social behaviour, while those who follow the other path will inquire into the instincts, sentiments, emotions, ideas, and beliefs of mankind, not only about strictly social events, but also about such events as birth and death which are of especial importance to society.

The two kinds of process, social and mental, are so closely connected that there must be relations between the two throughout. The two paths will have interconnections, even while they are parallel to one another, and these interconnections will become still more numerous as the paths converge.

A prominent cause of interconnection is the necessity, to which nearly every science is subject, of making assumptions belonging to the domain of another science. Both sociology and social psychology are subject to this necessity, and especially will sociology be driven to make assumptions which belong to the domain of psychology. In the older sciences, such assumptions are often well-established truths and can be accepted with confidence. The special feature of the relation between sociology and social psychology is that the assumptions borrowed by one science from the other can only be hypotheses, the validity of which is to be tested by finding how far they lead to the construction of consistent and coherent schemes. If these assumptions are thus justified, they become explanations. The point on which I wish to insist is that we must not mistake assumption for explanation. It is the danger of this mistake which makes so necessary the methodological separation of sociology and social psychology. It is just because it is at present so difficult to distinguish between cause and effect that each science should at present be followed so far as possible as though it were an independent discipline.

My position can be stated very briefly and in words of the utmost simplicity. I suggest that it is the business of sociology to ascertain what happens and what has happened before it tries to explain why it happens and has happened.

This proposition has two parts, referring to the present and the past. It might be thought that the first part would be accepted by all without question, and I believe it would be so accepted if the proposition were always put in the simple language in which I have stated it. And yet there is a vast amount of so-called sociology which consists of arguments that social events follow a certain course because our knowledge of the human mind shows that they must follow this course.

About the second part of my thesis there is a more serious difference of opinion, and I acknowledge at once that those who object to the necessity of ascertaining what has happened before we attempt to explain why it happened have some good grounds for their objection.

It may be said, and with especial force where societies devoid of all written records are concerned, that the chief instrument for the study of past history is a knowledge of psychology; that only through the knowledge of man's mental processes can we ever hope to reconstruct the past, so that the study of these mental processes should be our first care. I recognize the abstract validity of the plea; I have even a certain amount of sympathy with it, but it is my special object in this place to show that this is not the path by which we may hope most speedily and most surely to reach our goal. In the lectures on " Kinship and Social Organization," to which I have already referred, I have tried to show that certain social processes have been strictly determined, both in their general character and in their details, by social conditions, and that certain psychological processes which have been believed to be the determining factors are wholly inadequate to explain how existing conditions have come into being. The processes with which I was then dealing belong to the domain of social organization in the strictest sense, and it remains possible that, even if my contention were true of these, it need not be true of social processes of other kinds.

The lectures in question were followed by a discussion, in which Professor Westermarck was good enough to take the part of a vigorous opponent of my position. On one occasion, choosing an example of a social process which seemed to him incapable of any other than a psychological explanation, he asked : " How can you explain the blood-feud except by revenge ? " I propose now to answer this question, or, at any rate, to show the inadequacy of the answer which the form of the question implies. In Professor Westermarck's chapter on the blood-feud and allied social processes,[1] it is assumed at the outset that these processes are determined by revenge. The assumption seems so self-evident to the writer that he often speaks of the blood-feud as " blood revenge," and even uses this expression in the title of the chapter. After starting with this assumption, Professor Westermarck cites a number of cases in its support. He assumes that an emotion which explains certain actions among ourselves, and seems also to explain such a process as the vendetta of the Corsican, is also able to explain a number of cases from different parts of the world in which people take a certain line of action in response to a social injury. There is not a single example in the whole chapter of a case whose detailed analysis shows that either the general character of the action or its details can be explained by revenge. The assumption made at the beginning remains just as much an assumption at the end. The case is even

---

[1] *The Origin and Development of the Moral Ideas*, London, 1906, vol. i, p. 477.

less favourable than this, for it is evident that some of the cases cited by Westermarck cannot be explained by revenge as we experience the emotion, but only become intelligible on the assumption of a mental attitude very different from that which we adopt in response to a social injury. Thus, cases are cited in which the relatives of a murdered person adopt the murderer as a means of " retaliation " and treat him as one of their own children.

Melanesia provides abundant examples of the difficulty in explaining the response to social injury as actuated by revenge. A frequent cause of warfare throughout this region is adultery or rape. A community whose women have been thus injured makes war upon the offenders, and if this were all we knew, we might seem to have a definite example of the dependence of warfare upon the emotion of revenge. An inquiry into the manner of waging war, however, puts a different complexion on the matter. The people fight till one or more men have been killed on either side ; in some islands it is necessary that an equal number shall have been killed on each side. As soon as it is seen that each side has lost a man or men, the fight comes to an end automatically ; there is no parleying or arrangement of terms. Some time after, the two opponent peoples exchange presents which are of equal value on both sides. There is no question of the offenders giving a larger amount in compensation for the injury which was the primary cause of the quarrel. Moreover, ih the island of Eddystone in the Solomons, the party which takes the initiative in the exchange is not that of the offenders, but the order of giving depends on the drawing of the first blood in the fight. The side which first kills first gives.

It is, of course, possible that we have here only a case in which the workings of revenge are obscured by later con siderations arising out of rules of ceremonial warfare. Even if this be so, however, it is evident that revenge must take a far less important place in the social life of such people than it is supposed to take among ourselves. Revenge is a very inadequate motive to explain this form of Melanesian warfare.

The head-hunting of some parts of Melanesia bears a closer resemblance to the blood-feud in that two communities often take heads from one another over long periods of time. The heads are taken, however, for definite religious purposes, and there is no evidence to show that revenge plays any part in the process. The choice of a district from which to obtain heads is determined rather by the desire to obtain necessary objects as easily and safely as possible. A process which might seem at first sight a good example of blood-revenge is found, on closer examination, to be determined mainly, if not altogether, by certain religious needs in which revenge plays no appreciable part.

The method of which Professor Westermarck's treatment of the blood-feud is a fair sample is open to two grave objections. It leaves us at the end just where we were at the beginning in our knowledge of the blood-feud as a social process. I do not dwell on this objection because the book from which my example has been chosen does not profess to be a work on sociology, as I use the term, but on morals. We obtain from it no answer to such questions as the following : Is revenge a universal human character ? Is it an emotion which has developed or been modified in the course of the history of mankind ? Is it an emotion which has the same characters and the same content among all peoples, or does it vary with the physical and social environment ? An answer to one or more of these questions is suggested by some of the cases cited by Professor Westermarck, but he does not consider them from these points of view.

I have not made use of this example of the relation between the blood-feud and revenge merely as the means of criticizing the psychological method in general or its application by Professor Westermarck. I have chosen it because it seems to afford as good an example as I could desire of the true relations which should exist between sociology and psychology. Just as I believe that it is only through a detailed study of such social processes as the blood-feud that we can expect to understand the real nature of revenge and its place in the mental constitution of different peoples at different levels of development of human society, so do I believe that it is only through the study of social processes in general that we can expect to understand the mental states which underlie these processes. One of the chief interests of sociology is that it affords an avenue by which we may approach and come to understand a most important department of psychology. In place of asking, How can you explain the blood-feud without revenge? I would rather ask, How can you explain revenge without a knowledge of the blood-feud? How can you explain the workings of ·the human mind without a knowledge of the social setting which must have played so great a part in determining the sentiments and opinions of mankind?

The study which I have just undertaken supports the view that if he wishes to understand the social activities of man, the sociologist must begin with the study of the organized conduct which I hold to be the special province of his science. In plain language, it is his first business to find out what happens and what has happened. The processes by which this purpose can be effected are, however, far from simple, and involve problems concerning the relation between psychology and sociology which I have now to consider. To illustrate this subject, I propose to make use of an analogy which I have used on a previous occasion,[1] the analogy of

---

[1] *Sociological Review*, 1913, vol. vi, p. 304.

geology. We must remember that it is only an analogy, and, like most analogies, it may break down. I hope to show that this analogy breaks down and that the special point at which it does so is of the greatest interest to my main thesis. The analogy I propose to use is that the relation between sociology and psychology is like that between geology, on the one hand, and physics and chemistry on the other ; that just as it is the primary business of the geologist to determine the relationships and constituents of the earth's crust and the history of these constituents in the past, so is it the primary business of the sociologist to study the relations of social phenomena to one another in the present and their history in the past.

I shall now consider two aspects in which this analogy holds good in detail. One of these concerns the subject of definition. Though the primary task of the geologist is not to explain the relations within the earth's crust by physico-chemical processes, he may make use of physical and chemical terms in his definitions of objects and processes. Similarly, the view I put forward concerning the relation between psychology and sociology in no way precludes the use of psychological terms in the definitions of the institutions and processes of society. Such psychological terms may be used for two reasons. One, a matter of pure convenience, is that it is often possible to express by one psychological term or expression a number of social actions, positive or negative, which would take long to describe if all were enumerated. To give an instance : I have made use of the expression " to show respect for " in a definition of totemism.[1] " Respect " is a psychological term, but it is a convenient word which covers a number of acts, such as abstaining from injuring, killing and eating, which would make the definition cumbrous if enumerated in full.

[1] *Journ. Roy. Anth. Inst.*, vol. xxxix, 1909, p. 156.

The other reason which justifies the sociologist in using psychological terms in his definitions is that the sociologist has taken into his vocabulary a number of terms in general use which have definite psychological implications. If these terms are to be used at all, it is undesirable, or even impracticable, to deprive them of these implications. I may take such a term as " religion " as an example. Attempts have been made to deprive this term, as used by the sociologist, of the psychological implications which it bears in ordinary life. Definitions have been formulated which omit all reference to that belief in a higher power which takes so prominent and important a place in the concept of religion as the term is ordinarily used among ourselves. Two courses are open to the sociologist : one, to use a wholly new term, coined *ad hoc*, for the group of phenomena he wishes to class together ; the other, to use the word " religion " as we normally use it. In the present state of the subject, it seems best to use the current word, psychological implications and all.

The second aspect in which the analogy holds good up to a certain point is one which will take us into the heart of our subject. Though the primary task of the geologist is to explain the relations of different features of the earth's crust to one another in space and time, he has frequently to make physico-chemical assumptions, especially and significantly, when he is formulating mechanisms to explain how the various constituents of the earth's crust have come to occupy their present relations to one another. Similarly, the sociologist cannot do without certain psychological assumptions, and here, as in geology, it is when the sociologist tries to formulate hypothetical mechanisms by which social institutions and customs have come into existence, that he is driven to use assumptions drawn from psychology.

There is one department of sociology in which such psychological assumptions become indispensable, and it may perhaps be a convenient means of illustrating this aspect of the subject if I refer to my own scheme of the sequence of social strata in Melanesia.[1] The chief purpose of this scheme is to show how social institutions come into existence as the result of the contact and blending of peoples, how they emerge from the conflict between the culture of an immigrant and that of an indigenous people. One has only to think about the matter for a moment to see that the only way in which the culture of an immigrant people can be carried about the world is in a psychological form, in the form of sentiments, beliefs, and ideas. Immigrant people may carry with them a few weapons and implements, but even then the essential element which they bring to their new home is the knowledge of the way in which these weapons and implements are made and used. It is evident that the less material elements of their culture can travel in no other form. In formulating a scheme of the results of the social interaction between an immigrant and an indigenous people, we are therefore driven to assume the existence of sentiments and ideas possessed by the immigrants as the raw material of the process. Though the need is not so imperative in the case of the indigenous culture, it is convenient there also to assume the existence of such sentiments and ideas as will serve to explain the results supposed to have emerged from the interaction.

I have already pointed out that the geologist has to make assumptions drawn from physics and chemistry. So far the analogy holds good, but when we follow it a little farther we reach a point where it breaks down, and it is the point at which the analogy fails which I believe to provide so definite a support to the main theme of this paper.

The difference between geology and sociology is that the geologist takes from physics and chemistry assumptions

[1] *The History of Melanesian Society*, Cambridge, 1914.

upon the truth of which he can rely with certainty, while the psychological assumptions of the sociologist are largely or wholly hypothetical. The geologist can be certain that a million years ago, as to-day, water would not have flowed uphill and that heated gases would have expanded. He can assume with certainty that matter would have behaved in the way it does to-day at any epoch to which his imagination takes him. Can this be said of any of the psychological assumptions which the sociologist is driven to make? Is there any point at which he can affirm with certainty that man would have behaved, even a thousand years ago, exactly as he behaves to-day? Have we any psychological laws which can for one moment be put beside the laws concerning the behaviour of matter which have been reached by the sciences of physics and chemistry? I have never heard of them, and I am afraid I should not believe them if I had. It is just because no such laws are known, and just because I hope and believe that such laws can be discovered by the study of the organized conduct of man in society that I urge the priority of the study of social processes.

It is evident that the logical processes involved in this study of social behaviour as a step towards the discovery of psychological laws, are far from simple. In so far as it is the aim of the sociologist to contribute to psychology, his task will be the testing of his psychological assumptions. In so far as these assumptions enable him to formulate consistent and coherent schemes into which all known social facts can be fitted, schemes capable of explaining new facts as they are discovered, so far will the evidence in favour of the correct-ness of his assumptions accumulate. If, on the other hand, his assumptions lead to the formulation of unworkable schemes, schemes which will not fit with known facts, or, while explaining known facts, fail to explain the facts dis-covered by new investigation, the assumptions will have to be set aside, and attempts made to reach the truth by other paths.

I have so far considered the study of what I may call " pure " sociology as a channel whereby we may hope to attain knowledge of social psychology. This channel must necessarily be long and tortuous, and I must now consider why such a course is necessary, why we cannot follow the more obvious way of inquiring directly into the motives which actuate the conduct of men as members of society.

Among the people whose social conduct has been the special object of my own investigations, there is no more difficult task than that of discovering the motives which lead them to perform social actions. There is no more depressing and apparently hopeless task than that of trying to discover why people perform rites and ceremonies and conform to the social customs of their community. This is partly due to the abstract nature of such inquiries. In dealing with the concrete facts of social organization or with the details of ceremonial, the observation and memory of the man of rude culture are marvels of wealth and accuracy. Directly one approaches the underlying meaning of rite or custom, on the other hand, one meets only with uncertainty and vagueness unless, as frequently happens, the people are wholly satisfied with the fact that they are acting as their fathers have done before them. Thus, it would seem as if the people have never attempted to justify their social actions by the search for motives and meanings. When explanations are offered, they come from persons who have been in contact with external influences, and the motives assigned by such persons for social actions bear only too clearly the signs of this influence. They are merely the results of a rationalizing process used to explain actions whose sources lie beyond the scope of reason.

It may be argued that we fail to discover the source of

social action among such peoples as the Melanesian or the Indian, because we are dealing with modes of thought and culture widely different from our own and with people speaking languages which place insuperable obstacles in the communication of any motive they are able to formulate. Let us turn our eyes homewards, therefore, and see how the matter stands among ourselves. Such small experience as I have had myself in such inquiries has led me to regard the difficulty as even greater at home than among peoples of rude culture. If the task were laid upon me of learning to know the minds of people in regard to their social actions by means of direct inquiry, my own experience would lead me to regard the prospects of success as greater among such people as the Melanesians than among the inhabitants of an English or Scottish village.

Limited as is my own experience, it is fully in accord with all we can learn from those who have devoted themselves to such inquiries. The last few years have seen an extensive movement by means of which it has been attempted to gain knowledge, not merely of the social conditions of different classes, but of the mental attitudes which acts as the immediate antecedent of their actions. Those who have attempted such a task agree in their experience of its difficulty, or even impossibility.[1] They use language which might well be used of my own experience among savage peoples. There are those even who find the mental gulf dividing class from class of one nation even more difficult to bridge than that between the peoples of different nations taken as a whole.

It has in recent years been gradually recognized that social conduct is not directed by intellectual motives, but, predominantly, often it would seem exclusively, by sentiments or even instincts for which no intellectual ground can be assigned,

---

[1] See especially *Seems So !* by Stephen Reynolds and Bob and Tom Woolley.

which often seem even to run directly counter to the intellectual opinions of those whose conduct is concerned.[1] How often does one hear a man express liberal ideas, who recognizes himself that his intellectual sympathies are liberal, and yet when the time comes to vote, that is, perform a definite social act by which he can give expression to his ideas, he supports the other side. " Somehow or other," he says, " when the time comes to vote, I find myself voting conservative." If this position be granted, and it seems to be one which rests on very firm ground, the main thesis of this chapter necessarily follows. No mental states are more difficult to analyse than emotions and sentiments, to say nothing of instincts.

I should like now to call attention to a recent movement in psychology, a movement which, in spite of all its faults, I am inclined to regard as one of the most important which has ever taken place in the history of the science. This movement, which is connected especially with the name of Freud, not merely gives to the subconscious or unconscious a far more important place in the ordering of human conduct than has generally been assigned to it, but it puts forward a definite mechanism of the processes by which the subconscious or unconscious takes effect, and by which its workings are disguised.

I can only deal with this subject very briefly, and must content myself with referring to one process by which the activity of the unconscious mind is disguised, not only from others, but also from ourselves. I refer to the process of rationalization which provides rational, intellectual explanations of conduct that really depends on deeply hidden motives and unconscious tendencies to certain lines of action. Whatever may be the importance of subconscious or unconscious activity in the working of the individual mind, I do not think

[1] See especially *Human Nature in Politics*, by Graham Wallas.

there can be a shadow of doubt about its importance in what we may call the social mind. If Freud's views hold good of the social mind, they provide an ample explanation for the failure of those who have sought to learn the springs of social conduct by means of direct inquiry. That which we are told, when we ask for an explanation of social conduct, is but a rationalistic interpretation of behaviour springing from sources to which access can only be obtained by some indirect means.

The indirect means by which the subconscious activity of the individual mind can be studied are many and various. They include the study of dreams and the observations of the many departures from rational conduct (*lapsus linguæ*, etc.) which occur so frequently in daily life. Indications gained from these sources or from experiment may help in bringing to the surface of consciousness the hidden springs of action. Some of these methods have possible analogues in the study of the social mind. Thus, the myth of the social group has been likened to the dream of the individual. Mythology, however, is only an expression for one group of those social processes which, according to my thesis, open for us the prospect of a knowledge of the social mind. It is only by the study of such social processes and institutions as mythology, language and religion that we can hope to understand the mental states in which these and all other forms of social activity have their ultimate source.

It is of great interest that the Freudian theory should lead to conclusions agreeing so closely with those which workers such as Graham Wallas have reached quite independently and by the study of a department of human activity which, so far as I am aware, Freud has never touched. It is a remarkable fact that, through the study of hysterical nervous disorders, a physician should have been led to views concerning the nature of mental activity which agree so closely with those reached by the study of that branch of human conduct, also too often subject to hysterical disorders, which we call politics. Two widely separated lines of work have led to one goal and combine to show the importance of the unconscious and the misleading character of the intellectual motives by which the actions of mankind are usually explained. These two different lines of work in psychology support and justify the thesis that it is only by the study of sociology, in the sense in which I use the term, that we can hope to attain to a sound knowledge of social psychology.

II

FREUD'S CONCEPT OF THE "CENSORSHIP" [1]

In a publication [2] in which I compared the psychology of dreams with that underlying the rites and customs of savage peoples, I was able to point out several features of rude culture which present a remarkable resemblance to the rôle assigned by Freud to his endopsychic censorship. According to the writer, the unconscious is guarded by an entity, working within the region of the unconscious, upon which it exerts a controlling and selective action. It checks those elements of unconscious experience which by their unpleasant nature would disturb their possessor if they were allowed to reach his consciousness, and if it permit these to pass, sees that they appear in such a guise that their nature will not be recognized.

In sleeping, according to Freud, this censorship allows much to reach the dormant consciousness, but as a rule distorts it so that it appears only in a symbolic form and in apparently so meaningless a shape that the comfort of the sleeper is not affected. Or, the process may perhaps be more correctly expressed as a selective action which only allows experience to pass when it has assumed this guise.

In the waking state, the censorship is held to be even more active, or rather more efficient. It only allows unconscious experience to escape in the forms of slips of the

---

[1] Reprinted from *The Psychoanalytic Review*, vol. vii, No. 3, July, 1920.
[2] *Dreams and Primitive Culture*, Manchester, 1918. Reprinted from the *Bulletin of the John Rylands Library*, 1918, vol. iv, p. 387.

tongue or pen or to show its influence in apparently motive-less acts which, owing to the complete failure of the agent to recognize their nature, in no way interfere with the efficiency of the censorship.

There is no question but that this concept of a censorship, acting as a guardian of a person against such elements of unconscious experience as would disturb the harmony of his life, is one which helps us to understand many of the more mysterious aspects of the mind. Such a process of censorship would account for a number of experiences which at first sight seem so strange and irrational that most students have been content to regard them as the product of chance, and as altogether inexplicable. It is only his thorough-going belief in determinism as applied to the sphere of mind which has not allowed Freud to be content with such explanation, or negation of explanation, and has led him to his concept of the censorship.

There are many, however, prepared to go far with Freud in their adherence to his scheme of psychology, who yet find it difficult to accept a concept which involves the working within the unconscious of an agency so wholly in the pattern of the conscious as is the case with Freud's censorship. The concept is based on analogy with a highly complex and specialized social institution, the endopsychic censorship being supposed to act in the same way as the official whose business it is to control the press and allow nothing to reach the community which in his opinion will disturb the harmony of its existence.

Even though apparently close parallels may be found in rude forms of culture [1] as well as in the civilized societies from which the concept is borrowed, it would be more satisfactory if the controlling agency which the facts need could be expressed in some other form. Since the process which has to

[1] *Op. cit.*

be explained takes place within the region of unconscious experience, or at least on its confines, we might expect to find the appropriate mode of expression in a physiological rather than a sociological parallel. It is to physiology rather than to sociology that we should look for the clue to the nature of the process by which a person is guarded from such elements of his unconscious experience as might disturb the harmony of his existence.

It is now generally admitted that the nervous system, in so far as function is concerned, is arranged in a number of levels, one above another, forming a hierarchy in which each level controls those beneath it and is itself controlled by those above. If we assume a similar organization of unconscious experience, we should have a number of levels in which experience belonging to adult life would occupy a position higher than that taken by the experience of youth, and this again would stand above the experience of childhood and infancy. A level of more recently acquired experience would control one going back to an earlier period of life, and any intermediate level would control and be controlled according to its place in the time-order in which it came into existence.

Moreover, the levels would not merely differ in the nature of the material of which they are composed, the lowest level [1] being a storehouse of the experience of infancy, the next of the experience of childhood, and so on.[2] Much more important would be that character of the hierarchy according to which each level preserves in its mode of action the characteristics of the mentality in which it had its origin. Thus, the level

---

[1] I leave on one side for the present the possibility that there may be a still lower level derived from inherited experience of the race. If there be such a level, we must suppose that this is controlled by the acquired experience of the individual.

[2] It must be noted that in this concept the levels, like those of the nervous system, are not discontinuous, but pass into one another by insensible gradations.

of infancy would preserve the infantile methods of feeling, thinking and acting, and when this level became active in sleeping or waking life, its manifestations would take the special form characteristic of infancy. Similarly, the level recording the forgotten experience of youth would, when it found expression, reveal any special modes of mentality which belong to youth.

Higher levels of adult experience, then, acting according to the manner of adult life, control lower levels of infantile and youthful experience, acting according to the manner of infancy and youth. I have now to inquire how far this concept is capable of forming the basis of a scheme by means of which we may explain those facts of the sleeping and waking life which Freud refers to the action of his endopsychic censorship.

I will begin by considering dreams, the special form in which experience becomes manifest in sleep. The work to which I have referred, devoted to the study of the resemblances between dreams and the ruder forms of human culture, came to the main conclusion that the dream in its most striking form has the characters of infancy ; not so much that its material is derived from the experience of infancy, but rather that any experience which finds expression in the dream is moulded according to the forms of feeling, thought and action proper to infancy. This character of the dream finds a natural explanation if its appearance in consciousness is due simply to the removal in sleep of higher controlling levels, so that the lower levels with their infantile modes of expression come to the surface and are allowed to manifest themselves in their natural guise. The phantastic and irrational character of the dream is not due to any elaborate process of distortion, carried out by an agency partaking of a demonic character. It is rather the direct consequence of the coming into activity of modes of behaviour which in the ordinary state are held in check by levels embodying the experience of later life.

It will be well at this stage of the argument to state as precisely as possible how the view I now put forward differs from that of Freud. This writer supposes that his "censorship" is a process which has come into being as a means of protecting a sleeper from influences which would awake him. So far as I understand Freud, the distortion of the latent content of the dream is a result of the activity of the censorship. It is a transformation designed to elude this activity. I suppose, on the other hand, that the form in which the latent content of the dream manifests itself depends on something inherent in the experience which forms this latent content or inherent in the mode of activity by which it is expressed. If the controlling influences derived from the experience of later life are removed, the experience finding expression in the dream must take the form proper to it, and would do so quite regardless of its influence upon the comfort of the sleeper and the duration of his sleep. I do not deny that the infantile form in which unconscious or subconscious experience reveals itself in dreams may be useful in promoting or maintaining sleep, but if there be such utility, it is a secondary aspect of the process. It is even possible that this protective and defensive function may be a factor which has assisted the survival of the dream as a feature of mental activity, but the character of the dream is primarily the result of the way in which the mind has been built up. It is a consequence of the fact that early modes of mental functioning have not been scrapped when more efficient modes have come into existence, but have been utilized in so far as they are of service and suppressed in so far as they are useless.[1] I suppose that the general mode in which the mind has developed is of the same order as that

[1] Cf. *Brit. Journ. Psych.*, 1918, vol. ix, p. 242.

now generally acknowledged to have characterized the development of the nervous system, and that the special character
of the dream is the direct result of that mode of development.
As a by-product of this special development, the dream may
have acquired a useful function in protecting the sleeper
from experience by which he would be disturbed, but in his
concept of the censorship, Freud has unduly emphasized this
protective function.   His view of the endopsychic censorship,
with its highly anthropomorphic colouring, tends to obscure
the essential character of the dream as a product of a general
principle of the development of mind.

I can now pass to other activities ascribed to the censorship by Freud. The phenomena of the waking life which
need consideration are of two chief kinds.   Slips of the tongue
or pen, and other apparently inexplicable processes of forgetting, have been considered by Freud in his book on *The
Psychopathology of Everyday Life*. The other group which
needs explanation is made up of those definitely pathological
processes which occur in the psychoneuroses, for the explanation of which Freud has called upon his concept of the
censorship.

I propose to accept without discussion Freud's view that
such processes as slips of the tongue or pen are the expression
of tendencies lying beneath the ordinary level of waking consciousness.   My object is not to dispute this part of his scheme
of the unconscious, but to inquire whether such a scheme as
I have suggested may not explain these slips more satisfactorily
than as momentary lapses of vigilance on the part of a guardian
watching at the threshold of consciousness.

The special character of slips of the tongue or pen is that
a word which would be appropriate as the expression of
some unconscious or subconscious trend of thought, intrudes
into a sentence expressing a thought with which it has no
obvious connection, thus producing an irrational and non-

sensical character similar to that of the dream. If it is true, and that it is so seems to me to stand beyond all doubt, that underlying the orderly and logical trains of thought which make up our manifest consciousness, there are systems of organized experience embodying early phases of thought, and still earlier mental constructions which hardly deserve the name of thought, it is necessary that these lower strata should be held in some kind of check. Consistent thought and action would be impossible if there were continual and open conflict between the latest developments of our thought and earlier phases, phases, for instance, belonging to a time when, through the influence of parents and teachers, opinions were held directly contrary to those reached by the individual experience of later life. The earlier systems may and do influence the later thoughts, but the orderly expression of these later thoughts in speech, spoken or written, would be impossible unless the earlier systems were under some sort of control.

In so far as they are explicable on Freudian lines, slips of the tongue or pen seem to depend on two main factors ; one, the special excitation in some way of the suppressed or re-pressed body of experience which finds expression in the slip ; the other, weakening of control by fatigue or impaired health of the speaker or writer. A suppressed body of experience (" complex ") is especially, or perhaps only, liable to intrude into the speech by which other thoughts are being expressed when there has been some recent experience tending to call into activity the buried memory, while this expression is definitely assisted by the weakening of the inhibiting factors due to fatigue or illness. Such a process is perfectly natural as a simple failure of balance between controlled and con-trolling systems of experience, the temporary success of the controlled system being due either to increase of its activity, or weakening of the controlling forces, or both combined.

It is not so clear that it accords with the protective influence ascribed by Freud to the censorship. The slips of tongue or pen may be quite as trying and annoying as the suppressed experience out of which they arise. There is no such useful function as the guardianship of sleep which is ascribed by Freud to the censorship of the dream.

Another kind of experience fits better with Freud's concept of the censorship. The forgetting of experience when it is unpleasant or is a condition of some dreaded activity, of which such striking examples have been given by Freud,[1] definitely protects the comfort, at any rate the immediate comfort, of the person who forgets. The examples seem to fit in naturally with the concept of a guardian watching at the threshold of consciousness. At the same time, they are not immediately explicable as the result of a mechanism by which more lately acquired systems control more ancient ones of experience. They seem to involve a definite activity on the part of the controlling mechanism which is not inaptly designated by the simile of a censorship. In the case of the dream, I have pointed out that, if the scheme I propose be a true expression of the facts, we should expect that the controlling factors would sometimes acquire a useful function. This useful function need not be inherent in the process of development which brought the mechanism of control into existence. Just as there are certain features of the dream and certain kinds of dream which lend definite support to Freud's concept of the censorship, so the forgetting of experience which would lead to unpleasant action is a phenomenon which might be explained by the activity of a process similar to a censorship. Such a concept as that of the censorship, however, should explain all the facts and bring them into relation with one another. If it only explains some of the facts, it becomes probable that the process of censorship

[1] *Psychopathology of Everyday Life.*

is a secondary process, a later addition to one which has a more deeply seated origin.

The other group of phenomena of the waking life, for the explanation of which Freud has had recourse to the concept of the censorship, consists of the psychoneuroses, and especially that characterized by the mimetic representation of morbid states generally known as hysteria. A sufferer from this disease is one who, being troubled by some mental conflict, finds relief in a situation where the conflict is solved by the occurrence of some disability, such as paralysis, contracture, or mutism, a disability which makes it impossible for him to perform acts which a more healthy solution of his conflict would involve. The mimetic character of hysteria is definite, and the school of Freud has recognized the resemblance of the pathological process underlying it to the dramatization and symbolization of the dream. The disease is regarded as a means of manifesting motives belonging to the unconscious in such a manner that the sufferer does not recognize their nature and is content with the solution of the difficulty which the hysterical symptoms provide. According to Freud, the rôle of the censorship in this case is to distort the process by which the unconscious or subconscious manifests itself so that its nature shall not be recognized by the patient. This process is so successful that as a rule the patient not only succeeds in deceiving himself but also those with whom he is associated. On the lines suggested in this chapter, the concept of a censorship is in this case even less appropriate than it might seem to be in the case of the dream. The hysterical disability is amply explained by a process in which the higher levels are put in abeyance so that the lower levels are enabled to find expression. The state out of which the hysterical symptoms arise is one in which there is a conflict between a higher and a more recently developed set of motives, which may be summed up under the heading of duty, and a lower and earlier set of motives provided by instinctive tendencies. The solution of the conflict reached by the hysteric is one in which the upper levels go out of action, while the lower levels find expression in that mimetic or symbolic form which, as I have tried to show elsewhere,[1] is natural to the infantile stages of human development, whether individual or collective. The hysteric is satisfied with a mimetic representation as a refuge from his conflict, just as the child or the savage is content with a mimetic representation of some wish which fulfils for him all the purposes of reality.

The infantile character of the process is still apparent if we turn to the process by which the higher levels of experience pass into abeyance. It is now generally recognized that the abrogation of control which takes place in hysteria is closely connected with the process of suggestion. We know little of the nature of this process of suggestion, but there is reason to believe that it is one which takes a most important place in the earlier stages of mental development. If existing savage peoples afford any index of primitive mentality, this conclusion receives strong support, for among them the power of suggestion is so strong that it goes far beyond the production of paralyses, mutisms and anæsthesias, and is capable of producing the supreme disability of death.

This susceptibility to suggestion is to be connected with the gregariousness of man in the early stages of the development of human culture. If animals are to act together as a body, it is essential that they shall possess some kind of instinct which makes them especially responsive to the influence of one another, one which will lead to the rapid adoption of any line of conduct which a prominent member of the group may take. In the presence of any emergency, it is essential that each member of a group shall be capable of

[1] *Dreams and Primitive Culture.*

losing at once the conative tendencies set up by his individual appetites, and shall wholly subordinate these to the immediate needs of the group. Animals possessing this power by which the higher and more lately developed tendencies are inhibited by the collective needs set up by danger, will naturally survive in the struggle for existence. If, as there can be little doubt, man in the earlier stages of his cultural development was such an animal, we have an ample motive for his suggestibility, and for the greater strength of this character in the earlier levels of experience. According to this point of view, hysteria is the activity of an early form of reaction to a dangerous or difficult situation. The protection against the danger or difficulty so provided is the direct consequence of the nature of the early form of reaction, and the concept of a censorship, making it necessary that the manifestations shall take this form, is artificial and unnecessary.

The argument thus far set forth is that the phenomena, both of waking and sleeping experience, which have led Freud to his concept of the censorship are explicable as the result of an arrangement of mental levels exactly comparable with that now generally recognized to exist in the nervous system, an arrangement by which more recently developed or acquired systems control the more ancient. The special characters of the manifestations which Freud has explained by his concept of the censorship have been regarded as inherent in the experience which finds expression when the more recently acquired and controlling factors have been weakened or removed.

The concept which I here put forward in place of the Freudian censorship is borrowed from the physiology of the nervous system. I propose now to consider briefly some facts usually regarded as strictly neurological and to discuss how they fit in with the two concepts. In the case of the nervous system, two chief classes of failure of control can be recognized—one occasional and the other more or less persistent, at any rate for considerable periods. If the relations between the conscious and the unconscious are of the same order as those existing between the higher and lower levels of the nervous system, we may expect to find manifestations of nervous activity similar to those which Freud explains by his concept of the censorship.

Good examples of occasional lapses of control in the sphere of motor activity are provided by false strokes in work or play. The craftsman who makes a false stroke with his chisel or hammer, or the billiard player who misses his stroke, show examples of behaviour strictly comparable with slips of tongue or pen. From the point of view put forward in this paper, both kinds of occurrence are due to the failure of a highly complex and delicately balanced adjustment between controlling and controlled processes. If we could go into the causes of false strokes in work or play, we should doubtless find that each has its antecedents, and that the false stroke often has a more or less definite meaning and is the expression of some trend which does not lie on the surface. Such occurrences are readily explicable as failures of adjustment due either to weakening of control or disturbances in the controlled tendencies to movement. In the vast majority of cases, however, it would be very difficult, if not impossible, to force these into a scheme by which they are derived from the activity of a guardian who allows or encourages the occurrence of the false stroke in order to cover and disguise some more discomforting experience.

A more definitely morbid disorder of movement, which may be taken as an example of the more persistent class of failures in control, is that known as tic, a spasmodic movement having a more or less purposive character. This disorder is definitely due to a weakening of nervous control and is most naturally explained as a dramatization of some instinctive tendency called into action by a shock or strain. Thus, the tics of sufferers from war-neurosis may be regarded as symbols or dramatizations of some tendency which would be called into activity by danger, and the movements are often of such a kind as would avert or minimize the danger. The concept of a censorship is here not only unnecessary, but quite inappropriate. The form taken by the tic is that natural to an instinctive movement, but the tic depends essentially on weakening of the controlling forces normally in action. Its existence, like that of hysteria, or perhaps more correctly like that of other hysterical manifestations, may act, or seem to the patient to act, as a protection against prospective danger or discomfort, but it is probable that such a function is secondary. It is an example of the utilization by the organism of a reaction, the nature of which is determined by instinctive tendencies and in no way requires the concept of a guardian watching at the threshold of consciousness, or at the threshold of activities normally associated with consciousness.

I will now turn to the consideration of how far the process which I propose to substitute for Freud's censorship has any parallels in human culture, for since the control of one level by another runs through the whole activity of the nervous system as well as through the whole of experience, we should expect to find it exemplified both in civilized and savage culture.

Every kind of human society reveals a hierarchical arrangement, in which higher ranks control the lower, and inhibit or suppress activities belonging to earlier phases of culture. In certain cases this process of control includes the activity of a censorship by which activities seeking to find expression are consciously and deliberately held in check or suppressed. But this process of censorship forms only a very small part of the total mass of inhibiting forces by which more recently developed social groups control tendencies belonging to an older social order. When in time of stress the control exerted by more recent developments of social activity is weakened, the earlier levels reveal themselves in symbolic forms, well exemplified by the Sansculottism of the French Revolution and the red flag of the present day, but these symbolic or dramatic forms of expression are not in any way due to the activity of a censorship. They are rather manifestations characteristic of early forms of thought, by means of which repressed tendencies find expression when the control of higher social levels is removed. They are not distortions produced or even allowed by the social censorship, but are manifestations proper to early forms of mental activity which occur in direct opposition to the censorship. Censorship is a wholly inappropriate expression for the social processes corresponding most closely with the features of dream or disease, for the explanation of which this social metaphor has been used by Freud.

In *Dreams and Primitive Culture*, I have described certain aspects of ruder society which seem to show modes of social behaviour very similar to those qualities of the dream which Freud explains by the action of a censorship. I now suggest that these, like the censorship of civilized peoples, are not necessary products of social activity, something inherent in the social order, but are special developments. They seem to be specialized forms taken by the general process of control in order to meet special needs. It has been seen that the concept of an endopsychic censorship is capable of explaining certain more or less morbid occurrences in the waking life. A good case could be made for the view that the social censorship has in it something of the morbid, and that its existence points to something unhealthy in the social order. Whether it be the censorship of the press of highly civilized societies or the disguise of the truth found in the ritual of a

Melanesian secret fraternity, the processes of suppression and distortion point to some fault in the social order, to some interference with the harmony and unity which should characterize the acts of a perfectly organized society.

III

THE PRIMITIVE CONCEPTION OF DEATH

In recent years there has arisen in France a school of thought, led by Durkheim, which has given a new direction to those studies which deal with the earlier history of human society. One of my objects in this essay is to criticize the latest developments of the ideas of this school, and for this purpose I propose to consider the mode of conceiving death among people of low culture, and especially among the Melanesians, among whom I have myself worked. Perhaps the most convenient way in which I can illustrate in brief compass the leading ideas of the French school will be to describe their attitude towards the school of anthropological inquiry, which is now and has for long been dominant in this country.

According to the French school, the work of practically the whole body of English anthropologists suffers from the radical defect that it supposes social institutions to have arisen in consequence of the realization of primitive ideas logically kin to our own; that our social ideas have been moulded by long ages of the evolution which has produced our present condition of society, and Durkheim and his disciples reject the view that they have been operative at all stages of man's history.

Further, according to the French school, it is not only wrong to suppose that the psychology of the civilized individual can be used to explain social facts, and especially the facts of primitive human society, but it is urged that motives derived from the psychology of the individual state are out of place in such a study. It is claimed that social facts are of a special order, just as objective and independent as any of the other facts of nature, and require their own special mode of explanation. The members of the French school assume, and they have every justification for the assumption, that in early society there was a solidarity in the actions of men as members of a social group which gave those actions a quite specific character and makes it wholly illegitimate to suppose that they were directed by motives of the same order which actuate the individual, and they assert that the explanation of the facts of early society is to be sought in social conditions which have as their psychological correlative or expression what they call collective representations.

Durkheim and the other members of his school have made little attempt to formulate the psychological character of these collective representations, but in 1910 there appeared a book by Lévy-Bruhl,[1] which attempts to formulate the nature of these collective representations more definitely. Lévy-Bruhl puts forward the view that primitive thought is quite different from that of civilized man in two ways, one positive and the other negative. The positive character is that primitive thought is under the dominance of what he calls the law of participation, while negatively it is not subject to the law of contradiction which dominates our own thought and logic. It is with the second of these two characters that I shall deal especially in this essay, and I will content myself with only one example to show what Lévy-Bruhl means by the law of participation. This law is an expression of a large body of facts which indicate that primitive man did not possess the same category of individuality as we do. We analyse an object, say a human being, into various parts, his skin, his hair, his head, body and limbs, his internal organs, etc., and we regard these products of analysis as

[1] *Les Fonctions mentales dans les Sociétés inférieures*, Paris, 1910.

having a more or less independent existence, so that if we cut off a piece of hair it becomes a separate individual object. We have no idea of any necessary connection between the person and his hair, except that they once formed part of an object which we regarded as an individual. It is certain that primitive man has carried out a process of analysis similar to that of ourselves, but his category of individuality has remained different from ours in that he still believes in a connection between the parts of what was once a whole. The mere separation of a man and his hair, so that they come to occupy separated regions of space, makes them no less parts of the same individual, and, on the practical side, he believes that by acting on one part of the separated individuality he can act on the other.

This is merely one example, but it will perhaps illustrate the kind of attitude of which Lévy-Bruhl is thinking when he speaks of the primitive mind as being under the sway of the law of participation.

The other and negative feature of primitive thought, according to Lévy-Bruhl, is that it is not subject to the law of contradiction. Primitive man is not disturbed by what are to us obvious contradictions, and seems to hold, with apparently perfect comfort, opinions which are to us wholly incompatible with one another. I will give an instance from my own experience. During the course of the work of the Percy Sladen Trust Expedition to the Solomon Islands, we [1] obtained in the island of Eddystone a long account of the destination of man after death. We were told that he stays in the neighbourhood of the place where he died for a certain time until spirits arrive in their canoes from a distant island inhabited by the dead to fetch the ghost to his new home. On one occasion we were present in a house packed

---

[1] The facts recorded here were obtained in conjunction with Mr A. M. Hocart.

tightly with people, who heard the swish of the paddles of the ghostly visitors, and the sound of their footsteps as they landed on the beach, while for several hours the house was filled with strange whistling sounds, which all around us firmly believed to be the voices of the ghostly visitors come to fetch the man who had lately died.

Later, after visiting a cave at the summit of the island, we were given a circumstantial account of its ghostly inhabitants, and we learnt that after death the people of the island inhabit this cave. Here the natives possess two beliefs which seem to us incompatible with one another : if the spirits of the dead go to a distant island, they cannot, according to our logic, at the same time live in a cave on the island where they died. Of course the natural interpretation is that the ghosts live in the cave in the interval between death and the setting out for the distant island, or that while some went to the distant island, others take up their abode in the cave. It was clear, however, that the contradiction was not to be explained in these simple ways, but that the people held the two beliefs that the dead go to a distant island and yet remain on the island where they died.

I have taken this instance from my own experience and it is a good example of the kind of attitude which has led Lévy-Bruhl to assert that primitive thought is not subject to the law of contradiction. He has taken the two characteristics I have described as those of a special order of mentality for which he has used the term prelogical. The collective representations of the Durkheim school are held to be the expression of a prelogical mentality which is regarded as an early stage of thought distinguished by a collective as opposed to an individual character, and by the two special features which I have just considered.

Taking the primitive conception of death as my subject, I hope to be able to show that much of the supposed contradictoriness of primitive thought with regard to this subject is the result of a conception of death widely different from our own, and, that, once this difference is recognized, not only do the apparent contradictions disappear, but it becomes probable that the logical processes involved in the beliefs and activities connected with death differ in no essential respect from our own.

Death is so striking and unique an event that if one had to choose something which must have been regarded in essentially the same light by mankind at all times and in all places, I think one would be inclined to choose it in preference to any other, and yet I hope to show that the primitive conception of death among such people as the Melanesians is different, one may say radically different, from our own.

If any collection of words used by savage peoples in different parts of the world be examined, it will be found that each native word is given its definite English meaning, while many English words are also given a definite native equivalent. Often it is stated that the natives have no equivalent for certain terms of the English language, but rarely is any doubt expressed about the equivalence in meaning of the words that are given in the vocabularies of primitive languages. Thus, on looking up any Melanesian vocabulary you will find that some form of the word *mate* is given as the equivalent of dead, and that dead is given as the meaning of *mate*. As a matter of fact, such statements afford a most inadequate expression of the real conditions. It is true that the word *mate* is used for a dead man, but it is also used for a person who is seriously ill and likely to die, and also often for a person who is healthy but so old that, from the native point of view, if he is not dead he ought to be.

I well remember an early experience in the island of Eddystone in the Solomons when a man whom I knew well was seriously ill. I heard that he had been visited by a great native physician, who was shortly expected to return, and presently there came along the narrow bush-path the usual procession in single file, headed by the doctor who, in answer to my inquiries concerning his patient, mournfully shook his head and uttered the words " *Mate, mate.*" I naturally supposed that the end had come, only to learn that all that was meant was that the man was still very seriously ill. As a matter of fact he recovered. The oldest man in the island, again, was almost certainly over ninety years of age, and he was not only regarded as *mate*, though really one of the most alive people on the island, but in speaking to him people made use of an expression " *manatu*," which otherwise is only used in the religious formulæ of the cult of the dead.

It is clear that it is wholly wrong to translate *mate* as dead or to regard its opposite *toa* as the equivalent of living. These people have no categories exactly corresponding to our " dead " and " living," but have two different categories of *mate* and *toa*, one including with the dead the very sick and the very aged, while the other excludes from the living those who are called *mate*.[1]

Further, here and in my experience universally in low states of culture, these are not mere verbal categories, but are of real practical importance. Every one has heard of the customs of burying the living, customs well known to have existed in Melanesia, and I have little doubt that in the old days, whenever a suitable opportunity arose, those who were called *mate* would have been actually submitted to the funeral rites which would have made them dead in our sense as well as *mate*. Even to-day the Melanesian does not wait till a sick man is dead in our sense, but if he is considered sufficiently *mate*, movements or even groans will furnish no ground for abandoning the funeral rites, or the process of burial, while

[1] A similar condition seems to exist in the Polynesian island of Tikopia where, as the Rev. W. J. Durrard tells me, " life and health are synonymous ideas."

a person who, through external interference is rescued from
this predicament, may have a very unpleasant time, since it
would seem that nothing would make such a man other
than *mate* for the rest of what we call his life.

I cannot say positively that the Melanesian categories of
mate and *toa* are universal in low stages of culture, but I have
very little doubt that it is so, and the frequency of the custom
of burial of the living suggests their wide distribution. It
must be remembered that nearly all our stock of anthropological data has been collected by individuals, missionaries,
officials or others, who for their practical purposes want
the English equivalents of native words, and do not discover or
ignore such differences of meaning as those to which I have
just drawn attention.   I may cite the story—I am afraid
I do not know how far it is authentic—of the missionary
who was invited to a funeral. On joining the funeral procession, he could see no sign of the corpse, and on inquiry,
there was pointed out to him an old woman, whom he had
already noticed as quite the most cheerful and animated
member of the party. If he had inquired into the point,
I have no doubt that he would have found that she was
mate (or its equivalent), and that the object of the ceremony
was merely to carry out the logical consequences which
followed from the application to her of this term.

Such practices of burying the living have been definitely
used by Lévy-Bruhl as examples of prelogical mentality, and
therefore it would seem that he supposes such cases to be
examples of belief in contradictories ; that the people behave
as if a person could be at the same time both living and dead.
If he were to take up this attitude explicitly, it could at once
be pointed out that one term of the supposed contradiction is
being taken from a civilized category and the other from a
native category, but that if it were once recognized that the
natives have their own categories, which are different from

those of the civilized, there is not only no contradiction, but their proceedings become strictly logical. The burial of a person who is *mate* is the perfectly logical consequence of what I may call his *mate*-ness, and it would seem wholly false to label such customs as prelogical or to regard them in any respect as logically different from those of ourselves.

There is one further point to be noted which increases our tendency to regard such actions as irrational. We think of burial as a means of disposing of the dead body, but to primitive man it is possible—I believe even probable—that the matter is not at all regarded in this utilitarian way, but that burial or other means of disposing of the body is to him merely one of the rites suitable to the condition of what I have called *mate*-ness. One of the fundamental fallacies of the anthropologist, I would call it the anthropologist's fallacy if I were not afraid that it is merely one among many, is to suppose that because a rite or other institution fulfils a certain utilitarian purpose,[1] it therefore came into being in order to fulfil that purpose, and though it may perhaps seem strained and far fetched, I am quite prepared to consider whether even such a practice as burial, which seems to have so obvious and utilitarian a purpose, may not have really come into being from some quite different motive. However that may be, the special point now raised is that, whatever may have been its original cause, it is probable that to man in low stages of culture burial is conceived as merely one of a chain of rites designed to promote mankind from one stage of existence to another.

I suggest, then, that more exact and complete knowledge of primitive beliefs would almost certainly show that many of the instances brought forward by Lévy-Bruhl as examples of prelogical mentality betray no real contradiction at all, and no failure of logic in our sense. They are merely cases in

[1] Cf. *Man*, 1910, vol. x, p. 163.

which the facts of the universe have been classified and arranged in categories different from our own, and I now give an example to show that a Melanesian would probably come to much the same conclusion about ourselves which Lévy-Bruhl has reached concerning them.

There is no social institution which shows more clearly the existence of different principles of classification than that of relationship or kinship. In nearly all peoples of low culture, the whole system of denoting relatives is so fundamentally different from our own that we have no real equivalent terms in our language for any one of the terms used by them, while, conversely, such people have no terms which are the exact equivalents of ours. Thus, a Melanesian term which we translate father is also applied to all the brothers of the father and the husbands of the mother's sisters, and it may be to various other classes of relative. Thus " father " is obviously a wholly inappropriate rendering, and this applies throughout the whole circle of relationships. Further, the whole system of relationship plays an enormously more important part in the lives of the people than among ourselves. I hope the assumption will not be thought too grotesque that a group of Melanesians may, while preserving their own social institutions and beliefs, acquire a knowledge of psychology and logic.

Let us suppose that one of their number, fired with a desire to understand the mental processes of other peoples, sets out to investigate the condition of these islands. The extreme importance of relationship in his own community will naturally lead him to decide that the best way of procedure would be to study in particular our system of relationship as a means of understanding our psychology. He would soon find that we use terms of relationship in a way which to him is hopelessly confused and inexact. In studying the connotation of such terms as uncle and aunt, he would find that we include under these two terms relationships which he distinguishes very carefully. He would even find that we often apply the term cousin not merely to persons of our own generation but to those of older and younger generations than ourselves, betraying, it would seem to him, an almost inconceivable looseness of thought, so that he is tempted to suppose that we are not subject to the law of contradiction but believe that persons may be of the same and of different generations. He will return to his home and announce to his fellow-islanders that the English people, in spite of the splendour of their material culture, in many ways show signs of serious mental incapacity ; and that in spite of their fine houses and towns, their trains and their ships, their talking machines and their flying machines, they are the victims of the most appalling confusions of thought. It may even be that, at a meeting of the native Philosophical Society, he propounds the view that the hyper-development of material culture has led to an atrophy of the thought-processes, and suggests as a suitable title for the condition that of post-logical mentality.

I believe this is something more than a frivolous travesty of the mode of procedure which I am considering. I believe that my idealized Melanesian would be proceeding on precisely the same lines and making exactly the same kinds of mistakes as those who neglect the possibility that the apparent confusion and contradictoriness which they find in savage thought may be not in that thought itself, but only in their own conception of it.

I do not wish to imply a belief that all the obscurities to be found among savage peoples can thus be explained. As an example of a different kind, I may take the instance I have already given of the apparently contradictory beliefs of the natives of Eddystone Island concerning the abode of the dead. In this case I believe the proximate explanation of the contradiction to be that we have to do with a case of religious syncretism ; that the religion of these people is the resultant of the mixture of two cults ; one possessing the belief that the dead dwell in a cave of the island, and the other, the cult of an immigrant people whose dead returned to the home whence they came. I fully recognize that such a condition is not sufficient to explain the apparent comfort with which the people now hold these contradictory beliefs, but it seems to me to remove the necessity for any assumption of a radically different mental structure. The failure to attend to the contradiction becomes merely an example, partly of mental inertia, a failure to synthesize their religious beliefs ; partly, of a tendency to accept religious teachings without question and without attention to the consequences to which these teachings lead if followed out logically, a tendency which is certainly not confined to primitive man. Even, however, after such cases have been put on one side, it is probable that there will still be found others of real contradiction in primitive custom, but it seems probable that these are examples of a mental attitude which again is far from being limited to primitive people, and perhaps is not primitive at all. It seems not unlikely that this residuum of cases will be found to be of an order met with at all stages of human culture ; cases such as those of people who are perfectly happy in professions of belief on Sunday which their whole lives contradict on the other six days of the week. Yet such contradictions cause no mental discomfort or intellectual dissatisfaction.[1]

Even if the prelogical nature of primitive human mentality in Lévy-Bruhl's sense were established, it seems to me that the concept would furnish a very unsatisfactory working hypothesis for sociology. Prelogical mentality would almost certainly tend to become a convenient title wherewith to label any manifestation of the human mind we do not readily understand. The concept is like those of phlogiston and

[1] I must be content here with this somewhat crude example, for I do not wish to consider here how the general attitude of mind, which Lévy-Bruhl calls prelogical, is related to religious mysticism.

vitalism, concepts which have had much truth, but yet have provided, and in one case still provide, most dangerous working hypotheses. The adoption of the prelogical nature of human mentality as a working hypothesis would tend to draw away attention and effort from what I believe to be the fundamental duty of anthropology at the present time and for long times to come, viz., the discovery of primitive methods of classification and of the ways in which primitive man conceives the universe and himself. I am inclined, therefore, to think that in his book Lévy-Bruhl has taken a retrograde step. Some of the most valuable work of the Durkheim school has been in the study of primitive modes of classification,[1] and Lévy-Bruhl's own law of participation is of course but another attempt in this direction. It is not to this part of his book that I object. It is the stress he lays on the contradictoriness and illogical or prelogical nature of primitive thought which seems to me to be a step backwards in the work of his school.

I am afraid it may be thought that up to now I have said very little to justify the title of this discussion. I have merely taken a primitive way of conceiving death as the basis for criticizing a modern attitude to primitive thought. I have tried to show that much that has been assumed to be contradictory in primitive thought is the result of a certain manner of conceiving death, and I should now like to go a few steps in the direction which seems likely to show us the nature of this primitive concept.

The problem to be dealt with is the determination of the nature of the state which the Melanesian calls *mate*, the condition of *mate*-ness. The first point to be noted is that while with us death is an event which sharply marks off one durable state from another, *mate*-ness is itself a state, rather than an event, which may last for a long time, sometimes for years.

[1] See especially Durkheim and Mauss: "De quelques formes primitives de classification," *L'Année Sociologique*, vi, p. 1, 1903.

Next, it is clear that the two states which lie on either side
of this condition of *mate*-ness are to the primitive mind much
less different from one another than are the two states separated
in the civilized mind by the event of death. Even to the most
fervent believer in existence after death among ourselves, the
gap between life here and life hereafter is a great gulf. Death
is a sharp point of separation between two modes of existence
so different that few are able to form any clear conception of
that yet to be experienced, and with this difficulty of conception there must go a great difference in the sense of reality.
If it be claimed that both are equally real, it is clear that the
word ' real ' is being used in two different senses or in one
sense widely different from that of everyday usage.

To primitive man, on the other hand, I believe that existence after death is just as real as the existence here which we
call life.   The dead come to him and he sees, hears and talks
with them ; he goes to visit the dead in their home and returns
to tell his fellows what he has seen and heard and done, and
his story is believed, and he believes in it himself, just as fully
as if it had been an account of a journey to some country of
the living.   Further, life after death has the same general
aspect as life before death.   Thus, the Melanesian ghost eats
and drinks, cultivates and fishes ; he goes to war and takes
the heads of his enemies and, most striking fact of all, he dies ;
the life after death is not to be confounded with immortality,
which is a far later and more developed concept.   The second
point, then, is that the existence after death is as real to
primitive man as any other condition of his life, and that the
difference between the two existences is probably of much
the same order to the primitive mind as two stages of his life ;
say the stages before and after his initiation into manhood.

I may next point out that the life of primitive man is far
more definitely divided into periods than that of ourselves.
We have certain landmarks in our lives, as when we first go

to school or university or when we begin to earn our own bread, but such periods in the life of primitive man are far more clearly separated from one another. He does not gradually grow from boyhood to manhood, but he changes from the definite status of a boy to the definite status of a man by means of ceremonial which often lasts for a considerable time, it may be for years, and during the whole of this transitional period he is in a definite state or condition. There is a state or condition of a certain kind corresponding to the transition from boyhood to manhood, just as there is a definite state or condition corresponding to the transition from life to death, using these words in the English sense. Other periods of life are similarly accompanied by ceremonies which seem to indicate similar transitions from one state to another. In a very fascinating book, Van Gennep [1] has pointed out the general similarity between the rites which accompany the chief events of life, including death. In all cases there are rites which may be regarded as connected with the separation from the life of the previous state, while other rites·are associated with the transitional condition, and other rites again accompany the return to ordinary life in the new state, rites of reintegration, as Van Gennep calls them, into ordinary life. While the subject of the rites is in the stage of transition he has certain attributes which may be regarded as sacred, so that the rites of separation and reintegration may be regarded as rites of sanctification and desanctification respectively.

The important point to which I now call attention is that the rites connected with death would seem to have the same character as those accompanying various transitional periods of life. Taking Melanesia as my example, I might extend the conception of Van Gennep and suggest that the condition of *mate*-ness is the transitional stage ; that certain funeral rites are designed to promote the separation of the

[1] *Les Rites de Passage*, Paris, 1909.

person from the ranks of the *toa* and his assumption of the condition of *mate*-ness ; that other rites are associated with the condition of *mate*-ness itself, while other parts of the ceremonial of death are rites of integration into the ghostly life which is not regarded as widely different from life itself.

According to this conception, the passage from life to death is looked on by primitive man in much the same light and treated in much the same way as the passage from one condition of life to another. In order to understand the primitive conception of death we must study the ritual of death in conjunction with that of life. It would seem that the state of *mate*-ness is not something unique, but is merely one with which a man has already made an extensive and intimate acquaintance in other forms. To one who is not greatly affected by recent attacks on the doctrine of Animism, it will be natural to suppose that at these transitional epochs man is believed to be under the dominance of some spiritual influence, but it would take me too far to attempt any examination of the facts from this point of view. I must be content to have indicated the possibility that to primitive man death is not the unique and catastrophic event it seems to us, but merely a condition of passing from one existence to another, forming but one of a number of transitions, which began perhaps before his birth and stand out as the chief memories of his life.

IV

INTELLECTUAL CONCENTRATION IN
PRIMITIVE MAN

" THE chief intellectual difficulty of primitive man is concentration. He cannot keep his mind on one problem for
more than a minute or two." I had hoped that this belief in
the difficulty of mental concentration among peoples of lowly
culture had long been exploded. Apart from its incompatibility with all that we know of the strenuous conditions to
which early man must have been exposed if he were to keep
himself and his young alive, the statement is definitely contra-
dicted by all careful observation of existing lowly peoples. The
belief rests on the uncritical observations of early travellers
who found that the attention of the members of native savage
and barbarous races rapidly flags when they are questioned
about their customs. Such observations rest partly on the
wish of those questioned to avoid such inquiries, partly on
the fact that the inquirers have failed to arouse the interest
of those they have questioned, or have even diverted interest
by their obvious failure to understand the elements of the
matter they were curious about.

In my own inquiries into the beliefs and customs of lowly
peoples (including Melanesian, Polynesian, Papuan, Australian,
Dravidian and Nilotic African), I never found any lack of
mental concentration, once the interest of my informant
had been aroused, not merely in matters of perception and
memory, but where severe intellectual effort was required. On
the contrary, when the interest of Melanesian or Toda is once

awakened, it is I who have been the first to fail in mental concentration. Over and over again a conversation, sustained not for " a minute or two " but for three or four hours, has reduced me to a pitch of mental exhaustion and incapacity such as I rarely, if ever, reach as the result of the most complex conversations at home, my companion remaining alert and enthusiastic to the end, apparently ready to continue the conversation indefinitely. It may be objected that in such conversations I am trying to comprehend beliefs, sentiments and practices widely different from my own, and am seeking to fit together the pieces of a highly complex intellectual puzzle, while my informant is on his own ground all the time. On the other hand, it must be remembered that the rôle of my informant in such case is that of a teacher carrying out the most wearisome of all tasks, in that he is seeking to make another understand matters which seem quite clear and simple to himself.

A good illustration is provided by researches into genealogy. A large part of my ethnological work consisted in the collection of pedigrees and their employment as a means of acquiring social data. Two or three hours of such work have often reduced me, literally as well as metaphorically, to exhaustion, while my informant sat smiling and alert before me, apparently ready to go on with the topic for ever. I was fortified by the arts of writing and reading, while my companion had to rely on the thoughts and images provided by his unaided memory. On the other hand, I was acquiring and trying to piece together data wholly new to me, while my companion was dealing with matters familiar to him from childhood. But the methods I employed in such investigations often required much intellectual effort on the part of my informant, and these inquiries show conclusively that, once interest has been aroused, there is no difficulty in sustaining intellectual concentration for prolonged periods.

Summing up my own experience—and I believe this will be confirmed by anyone who has used the methods of modern ethnology—I may say that in intellectual concentration, as well as in many other psychological processes, I have been able to detect no essential difference between Melanesian or Toda and those with whom I have been accustomed to mix in the life of our own society.

PART II
PSYCHO-MEDICAL STUDIES

I

MASSAGE IN MELANESIA

WHEN I was working in the Solomon Islands with Mr A. M. Hocart [1], it was our custom, whenever possible, to accompany the native medicos on their visits to their patients. On one of these occasions the treatment consisted chiefly of abdominal massage carried on, so far as I could tell, just as it would have been by a European expert. On questioning the woman who was the subject of the treatment, I learned that she was suffering from chronic constipation, and if the matter had not been gone into more fully, it might have been supposed that the Solomon Islanders treated this disease according to the most modern and scientific therapeutics. Further inquiries, however, brought out the fact that the treatment we had observed was for the purpose of destroying an octopus which, according to the native pathology, was the cause of the woman's troubles. She was said to be suffering from a disease called *nggasin*, caused by the presence of an octopus in her body, and an inquiry into the diagnosis revealed the belief that the tentacles of the octopus would pass upwards, and when they reached the head of the patient, would kill her. The object of the treatment was to kill the octopus, and the treatment had already been carried out for several days, so that the octopus, which had at first been very large, had now become small, and was expected soon to disappear altogether. This result, however, was not ascribed so much to the mechani-

---

[1] As members of the Percy Sladen Trust Expedition.

cal action of the manipulation as to the formulæ and other features of the treatment which accompanied the massage.

On another occasion I observed the treatment of a case of supra-orbital neuralgia. The brow was kneaded carefully for a time and then a fold of the skin was caught and a motion made as though something were being drawn through the skin. The invisible object called *tagosoro* was thus extracted and blown away. I asked the leech [1] to carry out the treatment for *tagosoro* on my own forearm, and kneading manipulations, exactly like those of our own massage, were carried out till, by a sudden movement he showed me how he would have caught the *tagosoro* if it had been there, and would have blown it away. Here again a superficial inquiry would have seemed to show the existence of a massage indistinguishable from our own, and applied to conditions to which, according to our ideas, it is well adapted. It was only through systematic inquiry that it was discovered that the ideas underlying the treatment were wholly different from our own, and that the whole process rested upon a magico-religious basis. My object in describing this feature of Melanesian therapeutics is as an example of a difficulty which confronts that department of the history of Medicine which attempts to deal with origins. A few years ago I should have had no hesitation in regarding this Melanesian practice as an example of the growth of a rational therapeutical measure out of a magical or religious rite. I should have supposed that the practices of the Solomon Islanders were originally designed to extract the octopus or the *tagosoro* from the body, and that it would only be necessary to slough off what we regard as the superstitious aspect of the practice to have a true therapeutical measure. I should have regarded the Melanesian practice as one which has preserved for us a stage in the process of evolution whereby

---

[1] Mr Hocart has suggested that this old word should be used as a technical term for the practitioners of the rude art, which can be called neither medicine nor magic, but lies somewhere between the two.

medicine evolved out of magic and, as a matter of fact, I believe that the vast majority of my anthropological colleagues, at any rate in this country, would still be fully satisfied with this view.

Many students of anthropology, however, are coming to see that human institutions have not had so simple a history as this view implies, and that many of the cases, formerly supposed to show stages in a process of a simple and direct evolution, are rather the outcome of the blending of peoples and their cultures. The example I have described will show the possibility that Melanesian massage, as we now find it, may have had a very different history. It is possible that massage, much in the form in which it is found among ourselves and so many other peoples of the earth, was introduced into Melanesia by an immigrant people, and that the beliefs in the octopus or the *tagosoro* are merely the outcome of attempts to account for the success of the new treatment on lines suggested by the pathological ideas of the indigenous people. The process would be like that among ourselves when any new treatment, if sufficiently successful to attract attention, is explained according to the current pathology and therapeutics of the day. A case analogous to that of my Melanesian example would be the orthodox explanation of the success of Christian Science based on the pathological distinction between organic and functional diseases and the therapeutical ideas summed up in the term " suggestion." Before we accept Melanesian massage as an example showing us a stage in the evolution of a medical remedy out of a magico-religious rite, it is necessary to suggest the alternative hypothesis that it may have been the result of a blend between an introduced therapeutical measure and an indigenous belief. According to this, disease is due to animals or other agents which have found their way into the human body.

I cannot attempt here to deal fully with the evidence

which would enable us to weigh the two hypotheses against one another, for the subject can only be treated adequately in conjunction with the study of many other features of culture. I can now point only to two considerations. One is that true massage, such as is practised by ourselves, apparently exists in Polynesia. It is, of course, possible that deeper inquiry would show that, underlying Polynesian massage, there are ideas which give it a special character, just as we found to be the case with the massage of the Solomon Islands. But the way in which the Polynesians use massage as a restorative suggests that the massage of this people is a true therapeutical measure thoroughly comparable with our own practice. True massage thus seems to exist in the same part of the globe as the Solomon Islands. On the hypothesis of transmission, it may have been introduced into those islands by Polynesian castaways, who often found their way to the Solomon Islands, or more probably may have been brought to these islands by the same people who were responsible for its introduction into Polynesia.

A second consideration, to which it is very difficult to know how much weight to attach, is the extraordinary similarity of the massage of the Solomon Islanders to the true therapeutical practice. When I observed the massage applied to others and experienced its application to my own arm, the manipulations seemed to me to be like those of true massage rather than the result of an attempt to catch an animal or some less material agent. When we consider the intense conservatism of people of rude culture, their tendency for generation after generation to carry out operations in the traditional way, I cannot help feeling that the resemblance of their manipulations to those of true massage may be the perpetuation of the practice as it was originally taught to them, although the ideas underlying the practice have come to be very different from those of their teachers.

My object in this place, however, is not merely to introduce a curiosity nor to lay down any dogmatic view of its origin, but rather to point out a basic difficulty which confronts those who attempt to trace out the origins of medical beliefs and practices. Medicine is a social institution. It comprises a set of beliefs and practices which only become possible when held and carried out by members of an organized society, among whom a high degree of the division of labour and specialization of the social function has come into being. Any principles and methods found to be of value in the study of social institutions in general cannot be ignored by the historian of medicine. Here, as in other departments of human culture, the outstanding problem of to-day is to determine how far similar practices in different parts of the world have arisen independently, and how far they are the outcome of transmission from people to people. The fundamental importance of this problem is at last adequately recognized by the student of human culture, and I have ventured to use Melanesian massage as a means of calling attention to a problem which must be faced by all who attempt to study the origins and early history of medicine.

II

CIRCUMCISION, INCISION AND SUBINCISION

THE complex relations of medicine and religion are well illustrated by mutilations of the male genital organs, of which circumcision is the most familiar to ourselves. The mutilations take three forms : circumcision, in which the prepuce or a large portion of it is removed ; incision, in which the dorsal part of the prepuce is slit longitudinally ; and subincision, in which the urethra is opened posteriorly for a portion of its length, sometimes from the perineum to its orifice. Other mutilations are performed sporadically, such as perforating the prepuce or fixing objects to it. I hope to show that the operation of subincision differs wholly in origin and nature from circumcision and incision.

Both operations have a very wide distribution and the two forms of mutilation are frequently practised in different regions of the same ethnographic province. In Melanesia, the usual operation is incision, but circumcision occurs among the people of the island of Malekula in the New Hebrides, usually known as Big Nambas, and among the Sulka of New Britain, while it was formerly the practice in Fiji, where it has been displaced by incision, probably as the result of Tongan influence. Elsewhere in Melanesia, we find practices which seem to be intermediate between incision and circumcision in that the longitudinal incision is continued laterally, so that the lateral portions of the prepuce form masses one on each side of the glans.

In New Guinea, the operation is unknown, unless we

include Rook Island at its eastern end, which should rather be regarded as part of New Britain. In Australia, circumcision and incision are widespread.

In Polynesia, incision is widely practised, the chief exceptions which have been recorded being Penrhyn Island, Manahitu, Niue, Rakaanga, Pukapuka, the southern Paumotu Islands and New Zealand. According to Friederici, the people who practise incision in the northern Paumotus are colonists from Tahiti, and if so, incision was formerly absent from the whole of this archipelago. Although incision is not now practised in New Zealand, there is some reason to believe that some operation of this kind was known to the Maori.

In Indonesia, incision was probably the prevailing operation. This operation is performed in Nias and among the Igorot of the Philippines. In other parts of Indonesia, circumcision is the practice, but it may be that this form of operation is due to the Mohammedan influence, which is widespread in the Malay Archipelago. With the exception of the Semitic population, neither circumcision nor incision are known as indigenous practices in any part of Asia, though in Japan and the Liuchiu Islands the foreskin is kept uncovered, this probably being often assisted by artificial means.

The circumcision of the Semitic people is of course well known. As the founder of two widely differing religions of which the practice is a necessary part, this people has been responsible for the wide prevalence of the practice in Africa as well as in other parts of the world. Incision also occurs, however, widely in Africa and this certainly belongs to a culture antecedent to the introduction of Islam.

The operations of circumcision and incision have been included by Elliot Smith among the practices carried by the megalithic peoples. If, as Elliot Smith supposes, these practices spread from Egypt, it will follow that incision was the earlier of the two customs, for it was practised in Egypt from the earliest predynastic times till the dynastic period, when it was supplemented by circumcision.

Having given this brief sketch of the distribution and probable history of the two practices, I may consider how they serve to illustrate the relations between medicine and religion. That there is such a relation is shown very clearly by the custom of circumcision among ourselves. This operation occurs among the general body of the population as a surgical and hygienic remedy, the frequency of which has greatly increased in recent years, while among a special section of the population, it is a strictly religious rite intimately bound up with its religious traditions. There can be little doubt that the recent increase in the frequency of circumcision in this country has been due, though perhaps only indirectly, to Jewish influence. The observation of the beneficial hygienic effects of the custom among the Jews has been a most important factor in leading physicians and surgeons to recommend the practice as a hygienic measure. We have here a clear example in which an introduced religious rite has had a definite effect in fostering, if not in producing, the use of the operation as a hygienic measure.

It is probable that this relation exists elsewhere ; we know that in the Mohammedan and Jewish religions, which have led to the diffusion of circumcision through the world, mutilation is a definite religious rite. We do not know whether this was also true of the earlier waves by which the practice was diffused, especially that of the megalithic people, and the problem must be left for future research.

In Oceania, where the practice almost certainly came from elsewhere, the operation has largely if not altogether lost any religious character it may once have possessed. Like the social customs of many parts of the world, it persists chiefly as a result of the beliefs and sentiments of the women who regard it as an indispensable preliminary to marriage. In this region, however, hygienic motives have played a part in its persistence, if not in its adoption. Kubary notes that most of the inhabitants of the Gilbert Islands, where the operation is not practised, suffer from phimosis. If this were true of other parts of the Pacific, it may have acted as a motive for the adoption of the practice. We can be confident, however, that this would only have been a subsidiary motive, and that, without a motive of a religious or social kind, it would not be so widely prevalent as it is now.

Subincision.—This mutilation is especially characteristic of Australia, where it is practised over a large region.

According to the traditions of the people, the custom was introduced by strangers coming from elsewhere, and appears from these traditions to have been later than circumcision, which was already in vogue at the time when subincision was introduced.

The operation has elicited great interest on account of its extraordinary character and on account of the apparent difficulty which it puts in the way of procreation : a difficulty which, according to the most trustworthy accounts, is far more important than might be supposed.

The operation has been regarded as partly the result of a deliberate attempt to limit the population, but with this exception I do not know that any explanation of this rite has been suggested. But I believe that it has usually been regarded as a development of the idea of circumcision, and an extension of the idea of mutilation of the genital organ of which incision and circumcision are more simple examples. It has generally been supposed that the operation is strictly limited to the Australian continent and, since this continent has been regarded as one of the strongholds of independent origin, ethnologists have been quite content to regard it as a wholly independent invention of the aboriginal Australian.

E

Father Schmidt, however, has already drawn attention to the presence of a similar operation in Fiji, where it has a definite therapeutical purpose.

According to Corney and Basil Thomson,[1] the operation is called *tokalosi*, and is especially frequent in the central parts of the island of Viti Levu. According to de Marzan,[2] it is very frequent throughout Viti Levu, being called *tiki sinu* in the district of Ba, and *taka* over the whole of the western part of the island, including Nerua, Nandronga and the western hills. The operation also occurs in Vanua Levu. A reed is passed into the urethra as far as the membranous portion, where an incision about an inch in length is made down to the reed, so that a fistula is formed. Blood flows abundantly from the aperture, together with urine which is evacuated by this opening. In some parts of Fiji the operation is practised on young men with the intention of preventing the occurrence of those diseases for which the operation is regarded as a remedy. In another operation, known as *tuya ngalengale* in some parts of Viti Levu, *tava basi* or *tava sei* in others and *bita vitavita* in Navosa, the urethra is completely opened from the membranous portion to the meatus. Much blood is lost during the operation, which is said to remove the evil humours of the body. De Marzan points out that the operation has no relation to circumcision and is wholly independent of it.

A similar operation was performed in Tonga, to which place it had been brought from Fiji. The Tongan *tokalosi* is closely related to what Corney and Thomson call it in Fiji.

In the Tongan operation, a reed is first wetted with saliva and is passed into the urethra so as to occasion irritation and the discharge of blood. If the discharge is very violent, a double thread is looped over the end of the reed before it is passed into the urethra. When the reed is felt in the perineum,

[1] *The Fijians*, 1908.
[2] P. J. de Marzan : *Le Culte des Morts aux Fiji* : Anthropos, vol. iv, 1909.

it is cut down upon and one thread drawn from the aperture, so that when the reed is withdrawn one end of the thread hangs from the meatus and the other end, forming a seton, from the opening in the perineum. The thread is occasionally drawn backwards and forwards, producing great pain and much discharge of blood. The operation was especially performed as a cure for tetanus, and two patients seen by Mariner were greatly relieved, one in two hours and the other in six or eight hours, both cases recovering. The operation is also performed for wounds of the abdomen with the idea that any blood which has collected in the abdominal cavity will be evacuated by the urethra. It is also performed sometimes for general debility, but usually in this case the reed is only passed into the urethra to produce irritation and hæmorrhage and no incision is made in the perineum.

Mariner [1] gives a much fuller account of the applications of the operation than we possess from Fiji. Since the operation came from this region, we can be confident that, even if the Tongans developed and extended the usefulness of the operation, its motives were similar in the two places. These motives are of two kinds. The operation acts as a counter-irritant and as a means of evacuating blood and possibly other bad humours, which are believed to be producing or helping to produce disease. It is a strictly therapeutical measure with no trace of any religious or magical sanction.

The close resemblance of the Australian subincision to the operation of Fiji and Tonga raises a problem of great interest. If these closely similar practices have arisen independently, we have to suppose that in this part of the world two peoples of rude culture have not only independently invented a most extraordinary surgical procedure, but that this invention was prompted by wholly different motives in the two places. In the one place, it is a method of curing disease, while in the

[1] *An Account of the Natives of the Tonga Islands,* 1817, ii, 254.

other it is a rite by which youths become entitled to rank as men.   Australia and Fiji are not very remote from one another geographically, nor do their inhabitants differ very greatly from one another in physical character.   The factors of space and time and difference of race which are usually regarded as objections to the process of transmission are not present here, while all that we know of the customs shows that they are not due to any similarity of mental reaction to similar features of the environment.   They serve wholly different purposes and are performed from wholly different motives. The hypothesis of independent origin here leads us into a tangle of absurdities and contradictions.   There still remain, however, two possibilities.   One is that the procedure of subincision belongs to the culture of a people who once occupied the whole of this part of Australasia, and that the practice has only persisted in Fiji and certain parts of Australia, under-going divergent lines of evolution which, in one place or the other or in both, has greatly changed its original purpose. Thus, it has now become a purely therapeutical practice in one place and a purely magico-religious rite in the other.   It might be urged in favour of this view that very similar skulls occur in Viti Levu and Australia, skulls which bear a closer resemblance to the ancient Neanderthal skulls of Europe than in any other part of the world.

The alternative hypothesis is that some migrant people, who practised subincision, either as a therapeutical practice or a ceremonial rite, introduced it into Fiji and Australia, and that, in the process of assimilation into the indigenous culture of the two places, it has undergone such transformation as now give it its wholly different purpose in the two places. The special form of this hypothesis which seems the most likely to be true is that a migrant people introduced the use of a urethra seton as a remedy for disease, and that this has largely maintained its original purpose in Fiji, while in Australia it has taken on the special magico-religious purpose, characteristic of the aboriginal Australian culture. Having wholly lost all trace of its therapeutic purpose, it has become a purely ceremonial rite. There still, however, remains the effusion of blood, common to the two practices, which, in the one place, is the immediate motive, or one of the motives, of the therapeutic measure, while, in the other, it brings this rite into line with many other Australian rites in which the effusion of blood plays so important a part.

This common feature brings the practice into relation with the measures already considered, in which the abstraction of blood takes so prominent a place. It adds another to a group of practices which suggest that the abstraction of blood for therapeutic and religious purposes are not two distinct and separate processes, but are the manifestations of a belief which seems to have been widely diffused over the earth.

In relating both the Australian and Fijian practices to the loss of blood, it may be noted that one of the conditions for which the operation is performed in Tonga is the injury which is believed to result in effusion of blood in the abdominal cavity. It is believed that the channel by which the extravasated blood can be voided is the urethra. It is interesting to note that a similar belief occurs in the Solomon Islands. In the island of Eddystone, a condition known as *mamandara*, a word meaning blood, is ascribed to the presence of blood within the abdomen, and it is believed that the successful treatment of this condition avoids the mingling of this blood with the urine and fæces. As is usual in this island, the disease is ascribed to the breaking of a taboo and is treated by measures similar to those which usually are applied when the disease is ascribed to the breaking of a taboo, though in some cases massage of the abdomen is also employed.

Eddystone Island lies between Australia and Fiji. It does not share the practices of opening the urethra with these places, but it shows the presence of beliefs concerning the causation of disease, and concerning the nature of its mode of recovery, which are closely similar to Tongan ideas. Eddystone Island possesses a belief which acts as one of the motives for the operation of *tokalosi* in Tonga, but the operation itself is not known. If the beliefs have a common origin, we must suppose that the operation for the relief failed to take root at the same time, a result which might be expected, in view of the difference in the nature of the surgery of the two places. In contrast with the surgical skill of the more eastern islands, the operative procedures of the natives of Eddystone Island are in general so rude and trivial that, if such an operation as *tokalosi* had ever been introduced, it is incredible that it could have survived in such uncongenial surroundings. It is possible that we here have only another instance of the disappearance of a therapeutic practice when introduced among a people whose culture is dominated by religion.

III

SEXUAL RELATIONS AND MARRIAGE IN
EDDYSTONE ISLAND OF THE SOLOMONS

THE most striking feature of the regulations of Eddystone Island concerning sexual matters is the contrast between the great freedom before marriage with the great strictness afterwards. Soon after puberty defloration of a more or less ceremonial character takes place ; and this is followed by a period in which the girl is at the service of any man on payment of a fee to her parents. Once married, however, the rule is absolutely strict, though no doubt it is sometimes broken, that neither man nor woman may seek other partners.

Defloration is called *vanyoro* or *vari vanyoro*, and a virgin is called *katinyaro*. The defloration takes place at no very definite interval after puberty ; and it is clear that at present and in recent times it may be dispensed with, and a woman remain a virgin till marriage : but this is probably very exceptional and almost certainly unknown in the past. The matter is often arranged before menstruation has begun, and in such a case the man will give a ring to the parents of the girl in order to bind the transaction. Sometimes the girl has a voice in the decision, and the man chosen is one to whom she has taken a fancy. The regular fee for defloration is ten rings paid by the man to the parents of the girl. Usually, it would appear, one of the rings should be a *poata*.[1] This payment entitles the man to intercourse for twenty nights : but

---

[1] A kind of arm-ring.

if the girl is found not to be intact, the man will demand to have the rings returned and will only give the one *mbokalo* [1] which he would have paid in the ordinary way.

The defloration must take place at night and in the bush. Often the man is assisted by his friends, and it was said that as many as five might take part : but no actual case could be discovered in which there had been more than three. It seemed to lie entirely at the discretion of the man whether he should act alone or with friends, and the fee was the same in all cases, i.e. it would still only be ten rings even if three or more men took part. In such a case one man would go alone into the bush, and on his return to the house another would take his place. This continues every night for twenty nights, and then the girl is usually free for the custom which is called *varivosa*, according to which any man may visit her for two nights in succession on payment of one *mbokalo* or arm-ring. On these occasions intercourse takes place at night and in the bush. Never in any circumstance should inter-course before marriage take place in a house ; and there is some reason to think that if this did happen it would be regarded as equivalent to marriage, and the man would feel compelled to pay the marriage price. On the other hand, it was said that the pair might go to an unoccupied house. The rule about the time of day appeared to be less strict. It seemed clear that intercourse in the daylight was not absolutely forbidden, but there was evidently the greatest reluctance to perform it. It is definitely taboo for anyone after puberty to see the genital organs of one of the opposite sex : this applies also after marriage, and it is probable that the objection to intercourse in the daytime is connected with this taboo.

It was clear that intercourse sometimes took place before the more or less ceremonial defloration. About the time of our visit a girl had been found to be no longer a virgin and had

---

[1] A kind of arm-ring.

confessed to previous misconduct ; and in another instance a man said that he had been the principal in an undetected act. In relation to the former universality of this custom, it is probably significant that when a woman wears ear-pendants and other finery she is said to be *vavanyaro*. While a girl is subject to the *varivosa* custom she is a *vavanyaro*; and this seems to indicate that the condition was regarded as a regular preliminary to marriage.

A man before he has had intercourse is spoken of as a *komburu* or ' child,' even if almost adult, while afterwards he becomes *koleo*. It was said that a boy often remained continent till the age of eighteen or even older.

We did not learn from the people that sexual intercourse ever took place before puberty ; but a trader with a keen eye for such matters told us that he had seen a young boy and girl so embraced. It was quite clear to us that even at an immature age children were perfectly familiar with sexual matters, and the names of the genital organs were frequent in their conversation. This seemed to be recognized as more or less illicit, and these words were used in some measure in a prurient sense. For adults there is a strict taboo on the use of such words, and it would seem that they were allowed to be spoken by children, because what children did was not regarded as important. So with actual intercourse before puberty : it might be regarded as of little or no importance because the children were not responsible members of society.[1]

'It seems to be inconsistent with this report of juvenile

---

[1] We learnt that in New Guinea not only may sexual intercourse take place between children, but that little is thought of it even in the case of brother and sister, and in one example it seemed clear that a brother and sister were shown how to perform the sexual act by their parents. This happened in a part of New Guinea where incest after puberty is regarded as the gravest offence. Here it is clear that acts most clearly regarded as wrong when performed by persons after puberty may be looked on with a lenient eye or even encouraged before this period. These data show that there is no improbability in the statement of the trader which we record, though we did not obtain any such evidence ourselves.

intercourse that a boy might often or usually did remain continent till the age of eighteen or older. There seemed to be little doubt about this, and it is probably to be explained by the apprehension about sexual intercourse, which is an undoubted feature of early belief, intercourse before puberty being regarded merely as a form of play.

There was an idea that the first menstruation is in some way due to the influence of the moon. It is called *sa vagia na popu* or ' the moon makes it.' The idea was that the blood is the result of intercourse with the moon : but nowadays the people deny that they really believe this. They say it was used as a means of allaying the apprehension of the girl before defloration. The man would tell her that it was not really the first time, because the moon had already been with her.

Sometimes the defloration of a girl may be carried out by a native from another island, and at the time of our visit the daughter of a native of Mandegusu (Eddystone Island), who had lived for many years in Vella Lavella, was either brought to the island for this purpose, or the opportunity of her presence in the island was taken to carry out *vavanyaro*.

In connection with the dance and feasting called *vavolo*, many girls, called on this occasion *tugele*, were at the service, not only of the returning warriors, but also of visitors to the island. After a girl had acted as *tugele* she could no longer be procured in the usual manner, but remained chaste till her marriage.

An unmarried man and woman will sometimes go to the bush together without any payment having been made to the parents of the woman. This is called *vagalia ;* and the only penalty comes from detection, when the man has to pay. But it seemed that the anger of the parents would be appeased by a smaller sum than would have been given under the *varivosa* custom.

There are several regulations concerning this premarital intercourse. The brother of the girl should know nothing about the arrangements for the defloration of his sister ; nor is it right that he should know who has been with her or proposes to be with her under the *varivosa* custom. It seemed also that the husband should be supposed ignorant of the premarital doings of his wife, though he must often have been aware of them, for no secret is made of such matters. It was clear, however, that it would have been wrong to speak of the defloration of his wife before a man. It did not seem to be a strict taboo, but was more probably equivalent to our good breeding. The interest lies in the fact that it may be an indication of jealousy.

The most definite taboo of this nature, however, is between those who have been partners under the *varivosa* or *vagália* customs. A man may never mention the name of a woman with whom he has had intercourse before marriage, nor may the woman utter his name. Further, the two must not speak to one another, nor should they be in the same house together. In collecting the pedigrees, it happened several times that a man could not give the name of a woman, and in most cases it was due to this taboo ; and it was very striking to meet with this reluctance in a man of probably more than ninety years of age, as a remembrance of his youthful love affairs. The taboo on any kind of intercourse was occasionally a definite inconvenience to us, for one of our regular assistants might be unable to be with us if one of his former partners happened to be present. One man refused to hold the photograph of a woman with whom he had had intercourse before marriage. The restriction extends to widowhood, and a man who has been unable to speak to a married woman still labours under the same disability when her husband is dead.

Those between whom this restriction exists are *kenjo* or *kenjona* to one another. This is also the word for the process by which certain kinds of property are protected, a process which is certainly to be regarded as taboo ; and the use of this term seemed to justify us in regarding the restriction as to sexual intercourse an example of taboo, although it could not be discovered that an infringement produced any such definite consequence as it did with the *kenjo* on trees.[1] A difficulty is, however, introduced from the fact that a man and woman who have had intercourse are at once called *kenjo*, although this restriction does not begin till one or the other is married. It is possible that this is an extension of the term. They are people who will sooner or later become taboo to one another, and therefore they are called *kenjo*, even though the taboo has not yet begun.

Was Conception deliberately Prevented ?

The very free relations existing before marriage might have been expected to lead to the birth of many children and to the existence of definite regulations for assigning such children to their proper place in society. Such births seemed, however, to be extremely rare, and in the whole of the pedigrees collected by us only one such case was given, and that many generations ago. We did not hear of any such birth either during our visit or in recent times ; and so far as we knew there was no one on the island who was the child of pre-marital intercourse. It was said that such births occurred, however, though no actual recent instances could be given. Even if an unmarried woman became pregnant it did not follow that the pregnancy would be regarded as the result of one of the customs described in this chapter. For, according to the belief in the island, pregnancy may occur quite independently of sexual intercourse as a result of breaking the taboo called *kenjo surikai*.

It is quite certain that births before marriage were very rare, and two causes were given to account for this, abortion

---

[1] There is a reference here to other parts of his field work on the island. See, however, *Medicine, Magic and Religion*, pp. 32-33.

and a process resembling the other magico-religious rites of the island, called *egoro*, meaning 'barrenness,' which is believed to prevent conception. Abortion is called *junjui*, and may be produced by mechanical means, such as striking the abdomen with a stone, or by a process called *tambu njunjui*. In this rite a leaf called *meka* is heated and rubbed (*pua*) on the belly and four *tingi* leaves are held under the vulva, when, it is said, the child will come out. A girdle is put round the waist, consisting of a creeper of *boto na Vionona*, which has been lying across a path. The formula used when putting on the leaves is

" *Manjui pania na kumburu pini, ai ke tinoni.*"

" Take away the child here, may it not become a man."

The process called *egoro* is used before conception, when there is no question of a woman being pregnant ; and it is believed not only to prevent conception temporarily but to produce permanent sterility. It is even sometimes employed for this purpose before puberty. It may be used by both men and women.

Several examples of *egoro* rites were obtained. One came from Ruviana, in which bark is scraped with a *rikerike* from the two nut-trees called *ngari* and *vinu* and from the *petepete* tree. The bark is mixed with scrapings from a special reddish stone procured from the island of Gizo, and the mixture put inside a betel-leaf and given to the woman to be eaten with a nut of *anggavapiru* and lime, to the accompaniment of the following formula :

" *Ngge va pialia na rekoreko pini ; mi patu to pa na soloso ; mi ke pondu komburu ; mi egoro tu.*"

" I make this woman here eat betel ; let her be as the stone on the mountain ; let her not make a child ; let her be barren."

A girdle is put on of *molu* taken where it crosses the path. This is done for four months, once in each month.

Another method, elicited from a very old woman, was the scraping of bark from the *nggema* and *vino* trees. The bark was eaten with betel-leaf, together with *anggavapiri*, but without any formula. In the case of a married couple the mixture was eaten by both sexes, and it was said that, even if eaten by the man only, his wife would not bear any children. This rite was carried out for four months, four times in each month, and it did not appear that nothing was given on the third day of each period of four days, as in so many other rites. A case was mentioned in which this *egoro* had been given to a girl before puberty, who, though now a grown woman, had had no children.

This *egoro* bears so close a resemblance to the process already described that there are very probably two versions of the same rite. A third example is very different. In it, part of the nest of the bee or hornet called *mbumbu* and the flower of the *undundalo* plant are put inside betel-leaf and eaten with areca-nut, which is the *imburu* of the usual kind, while the betel-leaf is that called *uala igigisi*. No formula is used. This is eaten by men and women, and is said to be efficacious if eaten only by the man. The place of origin of this *egoro* is not known, and it may possibly have come from Ruviana like the first. The *egoro* rite has several interesting features from the magico-religious point of view, such as the likening of a barren woman to a stone and the use of a creeper which must have lain across a path. The chief interest of the rite lies, however, in the possibility that something may be used in it that has a genuine pharmacological action. It would seem probable that the efficacy of these rites is assisted by the regular use of some substance or substances which either prevent conception or produce early abortion. Any such substance must act by producing some pathological condition of the uterus, which when often repeated might produce permanent sterility. This sterility does not exist merely in the belief of the natives. The pedigrees show a very large number of childless marriages.

It will have been noticed that the *egoro* rite was sometimes performed after marriage, owing, it would seem, to the reluctance of the man to be troubled with children rather than of the woman to bear them.

Courtship

About the age of seventeen or eighteen, the young men begin to make themselves attractive to women and to decorate their bodies in various ways. They are then called *vavakoli* or *tinoni vavakoli*, while the corresponding name for women is *vavanyaro*. When a man or youth is *vavakoli*, he will wear arm-rings (*mbokalo* or *mbulau*), armlets (*tupatupa*) dyed red, and often similar leglets. In the armlets, he will often have scented leaves, and these are hung from the neck by a creeper. Two of the leaves thus hung are called *tanggala* and *riria*. The former is a large, almost transparent, yellow leaf with a pleasant scent, while *riria* is a resin. But the name is also given to a bunch of leaves of *ango* or turmeric, soaked in this resin. The leaves grow in Mandegusu, but the resin is obtained from Ysabel, often indeed the bunch of leaves already soaked, while the *riria* can now be obtained from the traders. They are worn both by men and women.

A man who is *vavakoli* will often wear a *torupai* or sunshade on his head, and it is doubtful whether this is now used for any other purpose. Both men and women wear ornaments in the lobes of the ears. In the old days, a *tinoni vavakoli* would also wear a stick, called *ogogotulusu*, thrust through the septum of the nose, and one or two of the eldest men still have their noses pierced, though the fashion of wearing the *ogogotulusu* had completely disappeared. Sometimes a group of young men, when *vavakoli*, would collect together and go about behaving like students in a rag, and once there was a general fight as the result of a party of young *tinoni vavakoli* cutting down some coconuts in pure mischief.

The initiative in proposing marriage seemed often to come from the women. If a girl takes a fancy to a man, she will carry off his basket and run with it to the bush, a custom evidently closely associated with that of the *tugele*, which is connected with warfare. Carrying off the basket is a definite sign of preference and, if the man is willing, he will begin negotiating with the parents of the girl. If he is unwilling, a girl may go a step further, and about the time of our visit, a girl, after having several times stolen a young man's basket, went one night to the house where he was sleeping. But the unwilling youth disappointed her by getting up and going elsewhere for the night.

If a man or woman is thus unwilling, attempts will be made to obtain his or her love by means of rites called *vakatapa*.

Love Charms

A number of means are employed to generate love in a man or woman whose aim is marriage rather than sexual intercourse. The process used has a general resemblance to the other magico-religious rites of the island, and is called *vakatapa*, *va* being the causal prefix and *katapa* a word which, on grounds already mentioned, may be translated ' love.' There were several *vakatapa* belonging to the island, while other very popular ones had been introduced.

One very simple form is as follows :

Four leaves each of *vonjamboe*, *irindi*, and *njorutu* are hung on a man or woman's neck with the words :

" *Nggoli vakatapa na mangota* " or " *na marani*," according to the sex of the desired one.

Nggoli is the name for the leaves collectively.

When the leaves have been put on a man, he goes to the

girl he desires and, if she takes hold of the leaves, she signifies her choice of the man and will marry him.   It is believed that this will always happen, but if there should be a failure in the action of a charm, it is ascribed to the failure of the girl to take hold of the leaves.

Sometimes, it appeared, the leaves of *riria* and *tunggala* might be added to or used in place of one or more of the above. All these leaves have a pleasant scent and are often worn, especially in the armlets and without forming part of any definite rite.

A *vakatapa* similar to this but more complicated was described by a very old woman, who had learnt it from her father.   It belonged to Ove, and at Nggema in that district there is a shrine in the form of a heap of stones.   In this rite leaves of the kinds called *vonjamboe*, *njorutu*, *irindi*, *vonjapoki* and *kenjokenjo* are hung by means of a *mamaroko* creeper on the neck of the man or woman who desires a mate, with the words :

" Mi ke katapa mi katapa tu na rekoreko ; mi ke mati mbola,
mi mbola tu ; mi ke mati kamu, mi kamu tu ; na leona, na rong-
gurongguna mi mati gua tu ; mi katapa tu pa na tininggu."

This may be translated :

" The woman does not love, let her love ; she does not want to come, let her want to come ; she does not want to come, let her want to come ; let her like his neck, his throat ; let her love by my body."

At the same time some moss (*lumutu*) is put inside the limebox of the man, and when he goes into the presence of the woman he wants, the latter will make use of his limebox, and by so doing consent to marry him.   But the mere sight of the leaves on the man's neck might be sufficient.

The names of a number of men and women who had obtained their spouses by means of this *vakatapa* were given.

One woman said that her father used to clear the shrine

at Nggema of overgrowth when he had given anyone this *vakatapa*, but he made no offering.

A *vakatapa* of a different form was given by a native who had learnt it from his father. In this, leaves of the *mboe* and *lembu* (mango) trees, the flower called *varu* and an eye of the bonito fish are put inside a betel-leaf and given to the woman when she asks for betel. No formula could be given and evidently none was used.

A *vakatapa* shrine was seen in Karivara near Kindawai, but the rite connected with it could not be fully revealed. It was said that a man who wanted to marry a woman took an areca-nut to this stone and after passing the night there conveyed the nut to the woman who, on eating it, would marry him.

All the above were rites belonging properly to Mandegusu, but in recent times two very popular *vakatapa* have been obtained from Ganongga and Ruviana.

At Ganongga, two leaves of *irindi* are put on a girdle so that they hang down over each hip ; a piece of *singosagi* creeper is put round the neck and from this one *njorutu* leaf hangs down behind ; a *singosagi* creeper is bound round the right wrist and shoulder-girdles of *aroso mbusambusa* are draped on each side. Most important of all is an outgrowth of wood which is called a *vakatapa* and is thrust in the basket. When the man goes into the presence of the woman he desires, he scrapes this *vakatapa* on one side so that the scrapings fall on the areca-nuts in his basket. The woman will ask for betel and he will give her nuts over which the scrapings have fallen. That night he will sleep in a house alone and if the woman has eaten the nuts, she will come to him there.

Sometimes the efficacy of the process is assisted by putting some scrapings of the bark of *anggavapiru* in the limebox and if the woman takes lime from the box, the charm will work.[1]

---

[1] See above.

Sometimes it happens that after having made these preparations, the man goes to the woman and she will not speak to him, nor use his nuts or lime. He will then eat some *piro* leaf and after that the woman will speak. No formula is used at any stage.

Although the immediate result of the success of this rite is that the woman comes to sleep with the man, it is clear that it is used when the man wishes to marry the woman ; indeed it was said expressly that it would only be used for this purpose, and many cases were given in which husbands or wives had been obtained by means of the rite. The wooden outgrowth called *vakatapa* is kept in the basket after marriage, and one was seen in the basket of a man who had used this rite to obtain his wife.

The *vakatapa* obtained from Ruviana was described by a native, who had learnt it from a man of that island on payment of a ring. His method was to scrape the bark of four trees, the *kate* (with an edible fruit), *lembu* (mango), *mboe* and *vetuvetugutana mao* and the scrapings of bark were put inside the limebox of the man who desired a woman, with the words :

" *Mana tu vakatapa pini, mati guania mangota ko ma ara via.*"

When the man goes to the woman she will use his lime and marry him. In some cases the man may obtain the woman's limebox on some pretext and put the scrapings of bark into it.

There is a regular fee for the use of this rite paid by the person on whose behalf it has been employed. In one instance the fee was not paid, although the man who had been assisted was successful in receiving his wife. The owner of the rite was angry, and spoke to his *vakatapa*, saying :

" *Sa ke venu na mbokolo, mule tu na nanggu vakatapa.*"

The *vakatapa* came back and the newly-married woman

no longer liked her husband and left him, although the latter
did not wish to part with her.

It was said that the *tomate* of the *vakatapa* took the scrapings of bark out of the husband's limebox and thus destroyed
the efficacy of the rite.

It will be noticed that the efficacy of most of these rites
is dependent on the person desired taking one of the materials
used in betel-chewing from one of the opposite sex. It might
be that a person would only ask for leaves, nuts or lime from
one already favourably regarded, but there is so much giving
and taking of these objects that there is probably little difficulty in transmitting the charm even without such partiality.
The fact, however, that accessory measures are sometimes
necessary would seem to indicate that where the purpose is
suspected, the objects will not be asked for or will even be
declined.

It is probable that the *tomate* of the *vakatapa* referred to
above is the *tomate* of one who had once known the rite, and
this idea is supported by the fact that some *vakatapa* have
shrines. In other departments of magic or religion there is
reason to believe that the shrines are the sites of old skull-
houses which had once contained the skulls of those who had
known and perhaps of those who had first introduced the
rites in question.

When a man has decided to marry a girl who has shown that
she is partial to him, he sends his brother or goes accompanied
by his brother to the house of the girl's parents, while the
brother arranges the matter with the father, who settles with
him the amount of the bride-price. If the father consents, the
bridegroom goes that night to the house of the girl and, after
presenting an arm-ring to her parents, passes the night with
her. On the following day, or soon after, he presents the
marriage-price, which consists of a certain number of *poata*,
usually ten, but only two for a widow, while as many as

twenty-five might be given for the daughter of a chief. Though the usual number of *poata* was ten, it was said that a man with a good reputation for industry might get off with less, and it is probable that there is a certain amount of bargaining, and that a man with a good position can make effective use of it in the negotiations. The presentation of the arm-ring before the first night brings the rite into the same category as the ordinary *varivosa*, and this ring is probably given so that if the man does not fulfil his bargain, he would then have paid the usual fee. In one respect, however, there is a clear differentiation between the first night of marriage and *varivosa*. In the former the man sleeps in the house, and it would seem that this was regarded as more or less of a marriage rite, and that a man who did not complete the transaction after having thus slept in the house would be looked at askance.

On the day following the marriage the man would go to work in the garden of his wife's parents, and would continue to live for some time with them, a residence in the wife's village that might continue indefinitely.

If the brother of the bridegroom who has taken part in the negotiations is quite young, he may be allowed to' stay in the house with his brother on the first night. Otherwise, he is given some food and returns to his home, while in the same way the girl's sister will not be allowed to stay in the house on that night unless quite young.

After marriage, neither men nor women continue to decorate themselves. If a woman were to do so, she would be suspected by her husband of trying to attract other men, and a man who continued to be *vavakoli* after marriage would be similarly suspected by his wife. Any *vakatapa* which had been used before marriage would still be kept afterwards, and would be believed to continue its efficacy in keeping alive the love of the partner who had first been attracted by its means. Men may also continue to wear scented leaves after marriage, but it was clear that this was only done for their wives' sake.

The *poata* given for a wife are not acquired by the bridegroom himself before marriage, but are contributed by the group of relatives he calls *taviti*, those to whom he is related by blood or adoption. Usually the man may be in a position to contribute one or more himself, but in several examples obtained nearly all were contributed by his *taviti*. When received by the parents of the girl, they are not kept by them, but are distributed to their *taviti*, so that the financial result of a marriage is the passing of a certain number of pieces of money from a group of people connected with the bridegroom to a group connected with the bride. It would seem not unlikely that this transmission of *poata*, which is no doubt carefully thought out beforehand, is a means of keeping ties of consanguinity in the minds of the people and of preventing marriages between even distant kin.

Adultery

From the moment that the ring is given on the first day, the woman becomes *tambu ;* she may not have intercourse with any other man, and even the mere suggestion of such an act might, if it became known, lead to a fight. This rule applies equally to the husband, and a lapse on his part might lead to a fight and would certainly be deeply resented by the wife. Such adultery is called *mbarata*, and a man who offends is regarded as *kunda* by others, this being a term which implies reproach. In cases of divorce, the restriction applies till the last *poata* has been returned. A woman may have definitely left her husband, but if the *poata* which he has given for her have not been fully returned, intercourse on her part with any other man would be *mbarata*, and would be as much resented as though she were still with him. That infidelity occurs under these and other circumstances is probable, but it is quite clear that it would have to be secret, and if discovered would meet with punishment.

This punishment is of two kinds, inflicted either by the injured spouse or his or her relatives or by the action of a *tamasa*. In the old days it was clear that adultery often led to fights, and its occurrence between a man and woman of different districts led to the definite fights which will be described under Warfare. In one case, a chief still alive at the time of our visit had killed a man because the sister of this man had committed adultery. The man who was killed had not apparently been implicated in any way in the offence, but was the victim of a vicarious punishment.

In addition to this punishment by human agency, there was a belief that adultery was punished in a more or less supernatural manner by *tamasa*, and especially by the shark, whale, and other marine *tamasa*. It was believed that a man who had offended would have his canoe upset and his body eaten by a shark (or crocodile ?). The being called Sea would also be angry with a man who had committed adultery and would kill or injure him with his club. Another supernatural intervention against adultery occurs in a rite carried out with the sacred *poata* of Mora. If any man present has committed adultery, rain will fall during the performance of the rite.

Several cases occurred about the time of our visit in which a woman who suspected her husband of infidelity had attacked and inflicted serious injuries on her rival. In one case at the time of our visit a native of the island suggested to a native from another island, who was in the habit of visiting the island and had married a Mandegusu woman, that he should have a girl brought off to his boat, and the suggestion at once led to a fight.

Divorce

The dissolution of marriage is a very simple matter, and is effected merely by the repayment of the marriage-price. The *poata* which have been given to the girl's parents have to be collected from those to whom they have been distributed and returned to the husband; and not till the last has been repaid will either party to the marriage be freed. When the *poata* have been received by the husband, he will have to redistribute them to those from whom they have been collected.

Cases occur in which a woman takes a dislike to her husband and leaves him. In such a case, it does not appear that the man has any means of compelling his wife to return to him. His only power lies in the fact that his wife can neither marry nor be the mistress of another if he declines to demand the return of the marriage-price.

The only motive given for divorce was dislike, whether mutual or on the part of husband or wife. Adultery appears to be only a ground for divorce in so far as it produces this dislike: but it did not necessarily follow, and in the few cases of adultery of which we heard, divorce had not followed.

Dislike of the partner to a marriage may be produced by a rite called *embi*, which may be regarded as a kind of reversal of the *vakatapa*. This *embi* rite is the possession of certain persons who will put it in action at the request of one who desires to separate a husband and wife in order to marry one of them.

Three examples of *embi* were obtained. One of these, in which four charred sticks are put inside the house of the couple it is desired to separate, came from Leoki and Njiruvidi. At nights the possessor of the *embi* stands on the left-hand side of the house (the *kali mairi*) [1] and throws on the roof-ridge

---

[1] By the left side of the house is meant the left-hand side when the man is standing inside the house with his face towards the door.

four unripe *ngari* nuts, and goes away, no formula being used. Next morning the woman will get up and leave the house without knowing why she is doing so, and will refuse to return to her husband. One of our informants had once produced this result with no other motive than curiosity. He had been taught the rite by a woman, but doubting the value of what he had been told, he went to the house of a couple chosen at random, carried out the rite, and he stated that the woman shortly afterwards left her husband, though he had no knowledge of the woman's dislike of him. In another example obtained from two widows, a small piece of turmeric was put inside a pudding. After a time the pudding is given to the man who wishes to part from his wife, and when he eats the turmeric he will no longer be able to cohabit with his wife. It appeared that this *embi* acted by making the husband impotent. The third example was similar to *vakatapa* and, like it, was obtained from Ganongga. Some scrapings are taken from the same outgrowth of a tree which is used in the *vakatapa*, but from the side opposite to that used in this rite. The scrapings are put, together with eight nuts of *nina*, in the basket of the man who is to be separated from his wife. That night the pair quarrel and the next day the wife leaves her husband.

It is interesting that the three *embi* are reputed to produce their results in three different ways : one, by making husband and wife quarrel ; another by producing the impotence of the husband ; and the third by producing an obscure impulse in the woman to leave her home. In all those cases in which the rite was performed with a definite motive, it was the woman who was desired by another : but it is probable that it may also be performed by or on behalf of a woman who wishes to marry the husband.

It appeared to be a matter of arrangement with which of their divorced parents the children would stay. If young,

they remained as a rule with the mother, but their relationship
with the father would be recognized and his *taviti* would be
the *taviti* of the children.   About the time of our visit, a man
had sent away his wife who kept the two children of the union
with her.   Later, she married another man who refused to
have the two children to live with him, and others took charge
of them, one, the mother's maternal uncle, and the other, the
husband of her mother's sister.   It is noteworthy that each
child was taken by a relative of the mother.   We could not
be sure whether this was exceptional, and due to some unusual
action on the part of the father, who had in the meantime
married another woman.   It was quite clear that if the
second husband of the mother had not objected, the children
would have continued to live with their mother.   One of the
children was a girl too young to have been named, a *tite*, and
it was evident that she would have received her name later
from the relative who had adopted her.

Remarriage

There is no obstacle of any kind to the remarriage of either
man or woman who has been divorced, the only condition
being that the money given by the former husband must have
been completely returned before the second marriage can take
place.

The remarriage of widows is less frequent.   Comparatively
few cases of such remarriages are to be found in the pedigrees,
and only one example could be given among people still living.
In the past, there was a case in which a woman was four times
married, the second marriage being with the man on whose
account she had been divorced from her first husband.   When
this man died, she married a third husband and on his death,
a fourth.   Another case was that of a woman whose husband
died after two children had been born.   A chief, evidently of

great influence in his day, wanted to marry her, but she refused and married another man who took her away from the island to Ganongga. Even there he was afraid that the chief would pursue him and so he left the island on a trading schooner, giving instructions to the people of the island to kill his wife as soon as he had gone, in order that she might not fall into the chief's hands. Both the woman and her son, at that time about eight years old, were killed. After being away from the island a long time, the husband returned to Mandegusu and married another woman.

Intercourse with a widow for the first time after the death of her husband is called *namboko vakarovo*, the latter word meaning "crossing" or "transference." This is *tambu*, or forbidden, though it probably occurs fairly frequently in secret. If discovered, the man has to pay one or two *poata* to the brother or other near relative of the dead husband.

The payment on marrying a widow is much smaller than for a woman first married. The usual price is one or two *poata*, which go to the woman's parents or near relatives. If, however, the woman has remained chaste during her widowhood, or is believed to have been so, a further payment is necessary to the representatives of the former husband. This payment will not be made if *namboko vakarovo* has already occurred, since in that case the payment will have been already made by another man.

Several regulations in sexual matters have already been incidentally mentioned. Further, it is regarded as bad form for men to look at women when they are bathing. At the time of our visit a man was in bad odour with his neighbours for having been caught spying at some girls while they were bathing. A man may speak freely of the genital organs of his own sex in jest, but he may not mention those of the other sex.

The Regulation of Marriage

Marriage is regulated entirely by kinship; a man is not allowed to marry a woman with whom he can trace any blood-relationship. A group of people connected by blood-relationship are known as *taviti*, and a man cannot marry his female *taviti*. The usual way of formulating the law is that *luluna* may not marry. This is the term given by a man to his sister, and reciprocally by a woman to her brother, and it is also applied by a man to all those women of the same generation as himself with whom blood-relationship can be traced, and this use of the term is reciprocated by the women. A man who is not permitted to marry a woman may not have intercourse with her either secretly or under the *varivosa* custom. No trace could be discovered of any clan or similar organization which plays any part in the regulation of marriage, nor did there appear to be any regulations prohibiting marriage between a man and woman of the same village. Cases were found even far back in the pedigrees in which this had happened, and the people were very positive that neither to-day nor in the past was there any restriction on marriage between two persons of the same place. Only three cases were discovered in which marriage had taken place between relatives and therefore contrary to the laws of the people.

One of these was the marriage of third cousins according to our terminology, both being descended from the same great-great-grandparent. The marriage did not take place in the ordinary way: for the girl was " stolen " by the man. Although the girl's father had been in no way responsible for the occurrence of the marriage, he had carried out a propitiatory ceremony in which a pig had been killed and divided into two parts. All the *taviti* of the pair attended, and the head-portion of the animal was given to the *taviti* of the husband and the tail-portion to the *taviti* of the wife. An areca-nut and a betel-leaf were also broken in two, and one half of each was presented to two groups of *taviti*. After this a *mbakia* and rings were put on the door of the skull-house at Ndaembangara, as an offering to the ancestors of the pair. In talking about the matter it was evident that though some years had elapsed, the girl's father had not got over the feelings of shame at the occurrence of this scandal in his family. The distant connection between the pair, so distant that among ourselves it would almost escape attention, had been the occasion for costly ceremonies and offerings and had left behind it a cloud on the life of the woman's father. We discovered another example of a consanguineous marriage among the islanders. Here the tie was closer, the pair being the children of half-brother and sister, i.e. of people descended from the same grandmother, but by two different husbands. Yet a third case cited from the past, but the pedigrees of these people were not obtained and their exact relationship remained unknown.

When a man first marries, he lives at his wife's village, and not infrequently remains there for many years, even for the rest of his life.

There seems to be little doubt that in the old days by far the greater proportion of marriages took place between people of the same district, and in such cases the pair, after going first to the wife's village, might go backwards and forwards between the two places.

When a woman had gone away definitely to live at the husband's home, it appeared that she thereby lost all rights to her father's gardens, while, on the other hand, a man living at his wife's home would have full rights to the use of her father's gardens.

Polygamy

Polygamy was in the old days a recognized institution of the island, and at the time of our visit there was still one man who had two wives. It was permitted only to chiefs and to those who had taken at least ten heads. Several instances were given in the pedigrees, or otherwise obtained. Thus, a dead chief of Simbo, who had two wives, had only taken five heads, but was permitted to possess his two wives because he was a chief.

One Simbo chief had taken twenty heads and had no less than eight wives. The capture of ten heads did not necessarily carry with it the possession of two wives, and the names of several men were given who had taken their ten heads but had only one wife. When a man had more than one wife, they lived in different villages and were visited in turn. The chief with eight wives was especially fond of two, and spent more time with them than with the rest. Clearly, there was often a good deal of jealousy. The present chief of Ove, for instance, first married a woman of Ganongga. When later he married a woman of Mandegusu, his first wife was angry and returned to her own island. It is probable that this jealousy may have prevented some of those entitled to the privilege from exercising it. The only man who had two wives at the time of our visit was not one of the chiefs, nor had he taken ten heads ; but he belonged to a family of chiefs and so was regarded as entitled to the second wife.

Polyandry was unknown, as was the institution of paramours found in so many places. But there existed a relationship between men and women, whether married or not, which suggested something of the kind, though it was said that sexual relations did not occur. The persons between whom this relation existed were called *mbaere*.

PART III

DIFFUSION

A.—PSYCHOLOGICAL

THE CONCEPT OF "SOUL-SUBSTANCE" IN NEW GUINEA AND MELANESIA

THE work of Tylor, Bastian, Frazer, and many others has acquainted us with the widespread belief that man possesses more than one soul, that his behaviour is governed by more than one agency of a spiritual kind which, to the rude intelligence, explains the thoughts and actions of mankind as well as the mysteries of sleep, disease, and death. The records which travellers have given us concerning these souls and their supposed properties, however, have been vague and scanty. As a rule we know little more than the fact that many peoples believe in a multiplicity of souls.

The Dutch ethnographers in Indonesia, and especially A. C. Kruijt, form a gratifying exception to this rule. They have collected a number of instances of native ideas concerning the spiritual nature of man. Among these ideas there stands out prominently one closely connected with man's vitality. Kruijt calls this animating principle *Zielestof*, or " soul-substance," but it is doubtful whether this term is the best that could be found. Most Indonesian peoples have the idea that this " soul-substance " resides in the living body and leaves it at death, when another spiritual entity, the ghost, comes into existence. For example, we learn from Kruijt that the Toradja of Central Celebes believe that so long as a person exists on earth he has a *tanoana* (soul-substance). Death is consequent on the permanent absence of the *tanoana* from the body. At the moment of death a double, called the *angga* or ghost, comes into existence and constitutes the post-mortem individuality of the person. Soul-substance and the ghost thus have different names and belong to separate categories of Indonesian belief. Moreover, the soul-substance persists after death, so that there is then a double existence, though only a single spiritual entity has been present during life.

The first point to be considered is how far the entity which Kruijt calls " *Zielestof* " corresponds with the " soul " as ordinarily understood. The evidence brought forward by Kruijt seems to justify us in speaking of soul-substance as a variety of soul. His account makes it clear that the term is used both for a more or less personal entity and for an impersonal principle or essence, with no hard and fast line between the two and with much of the vagueness of definition characteristic of the more abstract concepts of lowly people.

In its more personal manifestations, soul-substance can separate itself temporarily from the body during life. It may leave a person in sleep, dreams being believed to portray its experiences while away from the body. Its chief place of exit and entrance is by the anterior fontanelle, but it can also use mouth, nose, ear, or joint as its portal. If the soul-substance is away from the body for more than a limited time, the person falls sick, and if the absence is prolonged, he dies. It is believed that the soul-substance can be abstracted from the body, either by certain beings, usually termed gods, who dwell in the sky, by evil spirits, or by the ghosts of the dead. It is the business of particular persons, often women, to recover the soul-substance of the patient and thus restore him to health. These leeches, as they may be called, usually work by the aid of friendly sky-spirits. If the soul-substance has been taken by a sky-being, the soul-substance of the leech leaves his or her body and visits the sky in the company of the friendly spirit in order to demand from the god the soul-substance of the patient.

When the soul-substance leaves the body, it may assume the form of an animal, and in this state may devour the soul-substance of another person, who dies in consequence ; while if the animal in which the soul-substance is temporarily embodied is killed, its proper host will also die.

In all this there is nothing to distinguish the Indonesian soul-substance from the " soul " of many other peoples. I have now to consider a property of soul-substance which justifies the name applied to it. Soul-substance is believed to permeate the whole body and continues to reside in or adhere to any part separated from the rest, especially in hair, nails, teeth and the various secretions and excretions of the body. Since the sweat soaks into or adheres to clothes or other objects which have been in contact with the body, the soul-substance of a person can reside in or adhere to these objects. Certain parts of the body are held to be rich in soul-substance, the head, blood, bowels and liver being especially fortunate in this respect.

Animals, plants and inanimate objects also possess soul-substance, generally in the form of a vague, impersonal principle, but in some domestic animals and food plants it takes the more personal form associated with man, dogs, buffaloes and oxen being so favoured among animals ; rice and the coconut among plants. The consumption of anything possessing this form of soul-substance enables a man to add to his own store of the vital principle.

It is sometimes believed in Indonesia that the soul-substance is embodied in the shadow, but in this case it may be regarded as a " spurious " form of soul-substance. If a person's shadow falls on food, this should not be eaten by another, for the food will contain the soul-substance of him who casts the shadow. Soul-substance is also identified with breath ; thus in Nias, it is believed that a being who dwells in the sky has a storehouse of breath with which he vitalizes each newly-born human being, the breath again returning to the sky-being at death.

Among some tribes of Indonesia, it is believed that after death the soul-substance becomes the ghost, but this is the exception. The more usual belief is that the soul-substance goes to the sky to form part of a store from which newly-born human beings receive their supply. There appears to be a belief that one who receives the soul-substance of another resembles him in nature and is regarded as his incarnation.

The foregoing account is far from exhausting the properties ascribed to soul-substance by Indonesian belief, but it will suffice to give its leading characteristics. I should like to call attention especially to its intimate connection with life and health. In its more impersonal form, it would seem to be a kind of vital principle or essence. In its other manifestations, and especially in those where it has a more personal nature, it is not so clearly connected with vitality.

According to Kruijt, the concept of soul-substance underlies many beliefs and customs of the Indonesian. In its impersonal form it seems to provide the principle upon which sympathetic magic depends, being here combined with the belief that action on the part of the soul-substance is equivalent to action on the whole. The hair, nails or excreta of a person act as vehicles of the magic influence through the soul-substance they contain. Similarly, spitting is prominent in the treatment of disease because the spittle is the vehicle of the soul-substance of the leech. The bond of blood-brotherhood depends on the union of soul-substance consequent on the mingling of blood. The belief that a man acquires the characters of an animal whose flesh he eats, rests upon the belief that this flesh contains the soul-substance of the animal. A similar belief underlies both cannibalism and head-hunting, human flesh being eaten in order to add the soul-substance of the victim to that of the eater, while the heads of enemies are obtained in order to utilize the store of soul-substance which they contain.

The Indonesian beliefs which I have described thus provide a concept which links together customs of the most varied kind. Soul-substance may be regarded as a principle underlying the magico-religious beliefs and customs of the Indonesian, which is as comprehensive in its sphere as is our own principle of gravity in the explanation of the material universe. The customs which are thus referred to the working of a common principle are not special to Indonesia, but are among the most widely distributed beliefs and customs of mankind. We are forced to ask whether the concept of soul-substance is limited to Indonesia and is the product of the Indonesian mind, or whether it has a wider distribution, and underlies the magic, the medical art, the artificial kinship, the cannibalism and head-hunting of other peoples.

In a recent book [1], Mr Perry has shown reason to believe that the concept of soul-substance was introduced into Indonesia by immigrants who brought with them the cultural use of stone, the cult of a being connected with or residing in the sun, the belief in a home of the dead in the sky, and other customs, which he associates with the use of megalithic monuments. If, as seems certain, these immigrants came from the West, it becomes the task of the ethnologist to inquire whether, westwards of Indonesia, there is any evidence of a concept corresponding with the soul-substance of this region. To certain aspects of soul-substance there are clear parallels in the West, and I shall consider later the relation between the Indonesian belief in the double nature of the soul after death and the two souls of the ancient Egyptians.

Before doing so, I propose to inquire whether there is any evidence that the concept which Mr Perry believes to have been introduced into Indonesia has travelled further afield.

[1] *The Megalithic Culture of Indonesia*, Manchester, 1918.

If we go eastwards from Indonesia we come to two regions, Melanesia and Polynesia, which have so much in common with Indonesia in general culture, as well as in language, that their close relation is now widely accepted.

Moreover, it is held that this community of language and culture is largely due to migrations in which people have passed from Indonesia eastwards, and it is therefore an obvious and legitimate problem to inquire what evidence there is for the presence of concepts in Polynesia and Melanesia similar to that of the Indonesian soul-substance. I propose first to seek for such evidence in Melanesia and in the island of New Guinea that lies in the path of any travellers from Indonesia to Melanesia.

From one people of New Guinea we have an account of ideas agreeing very closely with those current in Indonesia. This comes from the Kai, a people of lowly culture and speaking a Papuan language, who live inland, but not far from the east coast of New Guinea. The account is given by a missionary, Ch. Keysser,[1] who was evidently acquainted with the work of the Dutch ethnographers, for he has adopted their term *Zielestof* in the German form " *Seelstoff.*" He tells us that the Kai believe in two distinct spiritual entities or principles, which he calls " soul " and " soul-substance " respectively, but he does not give their native names. The " soul " leaves the body at death to become the ghost, but has its own soul-substance, through which it becomes liable to vicissitudes, including its death, similar to those of its sojourn on earth. The " soul-substance," on the other hand, penetrates every living being and every object which we regard as inanimate. Every wooden object contains some of the soul-substance of the tree from which it comes and every stone the soul-substance of the rock of which it is a fragment.

---

[1] In *Deutsch Neu-Guinea*, by R. Neuhauss, Berlin, 1911, vol. iii, p. 111.

Soul-substance is contained not only in the hair, nails, excreta of a man, but also in his look, his name, and all his actions. The efficacy of the utterance of names in magical formulæ and of mimetic acts in ritual are believed to depend on this presence of soul-substance, which can be transmitted from one person to another or to an object, especially by contact. Measures by which soul-substance may be isolated are known, certain leaves being especially efficacious in this respect, and by this means a man can guard his own soul-substance or protect himself from the injurious influence of the soul-substance of another.

Another people of this part of New Guinea of whose beliefs concerning man's spiritual nature we have been informed, are the inhabitants of the small islands of Tami. The beliefs and customs of this people, who speak a Melanesian language, have been recorded by G. Bamler,[1] who seems to be unacquainted with the Indonesian evidence, for nowhere does he refer to " *Seelstoff*." He tells us that the Tami believe in two kinds of soul, which they denote by terms he translates " short" and " long." The short soul leaves the body at death and goes to the underworld of the dead. It, or rather the ghost which it there becomes, receives the offerings which are made to the dead, so that we can conclude with confidence that it represents the entity of the Kai which Keysser calls the soul.

The long soul, on the other hand, is identified with the shadow, and leaves the body to wander about in sleep, so that it resembles the more personal form of soul-substance of the Kai. Bamler says that the concept corresponds with our " consciousness," only personified. At death, the long soul leaves the body and appears to the relatives and then goes eastwards to the large island of New Britain. We are not told of any properties of the long soul which agree with those of the more impersonal form of the soul-substance of the Kai.

---

[1] *Deutsch Neu-Guinea*, vol. iii, p. 518.

In Kiriwina, one of the Trobriand Islands, at the south-eastern corner of New Guinea, the people distinguish two spiritual entities which leave the body at death. One called the *baloma*, which is identified with the image reflected from water, leaves the body at death and goes to Tuma, an island which, according to the belief of some, is connected with the nether world. Dr Malinowski,[1] to whom we owe this knowledge, was uncertain whether the *baloma* could be regarded as a soul dwelling in the body during life, or as a double which " detaches itself from the body at death." It is of great interest that Dr Malinowski should have been in such doubt concerning the state of the *baloma* during life, for if the *baloma* is a double which detaches itself from the body at death, the concept would correspond exactly with that of Indonesia. The other spiritual entity, called the *kosi*, is identified with the shadow. It exists only for a short time after death, frequenting the usual haunts of the dead man, such as his garden or water-hole. According to the belief of some, only those who had been sorcerers during life had a *kosi* after death, and another belief, also limited to some persons, was that the *kosi* became a *baloma* after a time. Since the *baloma* clearly represents the ghost of Indonesia, the *kosi* must be the representative of the soul-substance if the twofold nature of the Trobriand soul is related to the Indonesian belief.

The Mailu who inhabit the coast of south-eastern New Guinea from Cape Rodney to the middle of Orangerie Bay, believe in three spiritual entities.[2] Of these the breath is considered to be the vital principle which ceases to exist at a man's death ; the second is that spiritual part of a man which wanders to the nether regions when he dies, and the third is an entity which dwells in the severed and preserved skull. The prominence of the head as a vehicle of soul-substance in

---

[1] *Journ. Roy. Anth. Inst.*, 1916, col. xlvi, p. 353.
[2] B. Malinowski, *Trans. Roy. Soc. of South Australia*, 1915, vol. xxxix, p. 653.

Indonesia suggests that the third of these spiritual agencies may be the Mailu representative of the Indonesian soul-substance, but this is also identified with the breath, so that the Mailu have two beliefs which may be connected with the Indonesian concept.

The Koita and Motu believe in the existence of an entity, called *sua* by the Koita and *lauma* by the Motu, the absence of which from the body causes sickness. It is also believed to leave the body in sleep and to become the ghost at death. Among the Motu, pigs have a *laulauma* which comes to an end when the animal dies so that it has no *lauma* or ghost. The shrinkage in size of a pig at death is ascribed to the absence of the *laulauma*.[1]

Lieut. E. W. P. Chinnery records [2] beliefs of the people of the mountainous districts of Papua which bear a closer likeness to the Indonesian concept of soul-substance. The body is believed to be permeated by the " strength " of a " thing within," the influence of which becomes attached to everything with which the body is in any way associated. The " thing within " itself becomes the ghost after death, so that it would appear as if the concept of soul-substance has become an attribute of an entity within the body which becomes the ghost at death. The nature of the relation between the two is well illustrated by the belief that the status of a ghost depends on the " strength " of his soul during life. Various customs, including cannibalism and the anointing of the body with the juices of the decaying dead, depend on the desire to add to the " strength " of the soul.

If now we pass from New Guinea eastwards, we find that in one part of New Ireland the soul is called *tanua*, a word of which the primary meaning is said to be " shadow." It is regarded as a principle which gives life to the body and con-

---

[1] C. G. Seligmann, *The Melanesians of British New Guinea*, Cambridge, 1910, p. 189.
[2] *Man*, vol. xix, 1919, p. 132.

tinues to exist after death, being then called *tabaran*, the ghost of the dead. Peekel [1] says explicitly that animals and plants have no souls. The *tanua* of this region therefore corresponds with the soul of the Kai, and the only point of resemblance with soul-substance is its identification with the shadow. While the open religious cult of this region thus shows no evidence of the idea of soul-substance, there is much in common between this concept and the belief of the secret organization of New Ireland and New Britain called the *Ingiet*.[2] Members of this society can, if they wish, undergo a special initiation which allows them to take part in a rite called *e magit*. *Magit* is a term for something within a person which can be projected or ejected from the body so that it assumes, it may be the form of an animal, it may be that of another human being. When, as is usually the case, a member of the *Ingiet* projects his *magit* in order to do harm to another person, the *magit* becomes the vehicle by means of which the man carries out a process corresponding to the malignant magic of other peoples.

These beliefs in the existence within a person of a principle which can take the form of an animal and in that form act upon and injure another person bring us very near to the more personal form of the Indonesian concept of soul-substance. It may be noted that, while in New Britain and New Ireland the power of projecting the *magit* is closely connected with certain stone images, the concept of soul-substance in Indonesia is, according to Perry, closely associated with the cultural and ceremonial use of stone.[3] I might point out that it is quite in accordance with my own scheme of the genesis of the secret organizations of Melanesia [4] that they

[1] *Religion u. Zauberei auf d. mittleren Neu-Mecklenburg*, Munster, 1910, p. 14.
[2] See W. H. R. Rivers, *The History of Melanesian Society*, 1914, vol. ii, p. 515.
[3] *Op. cit.*, p. 153.
[4] *Op. cit.*, vol. ii, p. 205.

should have preserved, though in distorted form, features of an introduced concept which failed to implant itself in the beliefs of the people at large.

According to Geo. Brown,[1] the people of New Britain call the soul *nio*, which is also applied to the shadow. This soul leaves the body temporarily in sleep or fainting and permanently at death. Apparently it becomes one of the several kinds of being which are classed together as *tabaran*. Brown says definitely that there is only one kind of soul, but this can appear in many forms and enters into animals such as rats, lizards and birds. Animals have souls independently of this incarnation of the souls of men, but plants have no souls. Danks[2] also states that the spirits of men can enter into animals.

In the account given by Brown, which probably applies specially to Duke of York Island, the *nio* corresponds in several respects with the more personal form of soul-substance, but it is probable that it becomes the ghost and if so would differ essentially from the Indonesian concept.

In the Buin district of Bougainville[3] the soul is called *ura*, a word also used for shadow, reflection and dream. The *ura* leaves a man in sleep or illness and flies in the form of a bird to the underworld, where stands a tree, the leaves of which represent human lives. If the soul-bird plucks the leaf representing its host, the man dies and the soul-bird stays in the underworld. It may be noted that this appearance of the human soul in the form of a bird is associated in Buin with an unusually pure form of bird-totemism.

In the Shortland Islands,[4] the culture of which has much in common with that of Buin, the soul is called *nunu*. This

---

[1] *Melanesians and Polynesians*, London, 1910, p. 190.
[2] *Rep. Austral. Ass.*, 1909, vol. xii, p. 454.
[3] R. Thurnwald, *Forschungen auf d. Salomo-Inseln u. d. Bismarck-Archipel*, Berlin, 1912, vol. i, p. 316.
[4] G. C. Wheeler, *Arch. f. Religionswiss.*, 1914, vol. xvii, p. 86.

word is said by Wheeler to mean the lasting principle or essence of a human being and is also used for the shadow and the reflection. When a man dies, the *nunu* becomes a *nitu* or ghost, one cause of death being the catching of the *nunu* by a shooting-star, while some kinds of *nitu* also have the power of carrying off the soul. Defective intelligence is ascribed to loss of the *nunu*. In a case of this kind recorded by Wheeler, the *nunu*, though taken in childhood, was said to be still present and this apparent contradiction may possibly point to a duality in the concept.

In the Shortlands, things have *nunu*, and a ghost to whom an offering is made eats the *nunu* of the offering. A dead man also takes with him to the next world the *nunu* of the objects which are destroyed at his death. There is thus much in common between the soul of the Shortlands and the personal form of the soul-substance of Indonesia.

In Eddystone Island (which, though only about 50 miles from the Shortlands, differs profoundly from those islands in culture), the soul is called *ghalaghala*, a word also used for the shadow and reflection. When a man dreams, his *ghalaghala* leaves him so long as the dream lasts, and it leaves him permanently at death. The *ghalaghala* is said to be all over a man, thus accounting for the complete-ness of the reflection seen in a mirror. Things also have *ghalaghala*. When an object is burnt in the rites after death, its *ghalaghala* goes with the ghost to the place of the dead in Bougainville.

It is quite clear that there was only one word in Eddystone Island for the soul, but some of the death-rites [1] suggest the double nature of the corresponding concept. Soon after death a rite is performed in which the *ghalaghala* is caught and put under the ridge-pole of the house. While the *ghala-ghala* is under the roof of the house, a second ceremony

[1] I am indebted to Mr Hocart for the account of these rites.

takes place in which the *ghalaghala* is said to go to a cave near the highest point of the island. On the eighteenth day after death, the *ghalaghala*, although supposed to have departed, is transferred with the skull to a special shrine, while still later the ghost of the dead man, now called a *tomate*, goes to the home of the dead in Bougainville. This twofold nature of the destination of the soul points to its double nature.

Eddystone Island is the seat of a definite skull-cult, but there is no evidence that any spirit comparable with the head-spirit of the Mailu is believed to dwell in the head (see p. 104).

In Florida, the soul is called *tarunga*.[1] It leaves the body in sleep and after death becomes a *tindalo* or ghost. The only hint of a double nature is given in the fact that a pig has a *tarunga*, but this never becomes a *tindalo*.

In San Cristoval, Dr C. E. Fox records the existence of two souls which in Bauro, the home of the dual organization,[2] are called *ataro* or *aunga* and *nununa*, while at Wango, the point of junction between the region of bird-totemism and the dual region, the two souls are called *aunga* and *adaro*. The *aunga* of Wango is compared with the shadow caused by the sun and the *adaro* with the reflection in water. When a man dies, the *aunga* comes out either at the fontanelle or from the mouth, and sets out on its journey to Rodomana, the distant home of the dead. The *adaro*, on the other hand, remains for some time with the body and then goes either into the jaw-bone, into a small stone statue placed on the burial-mound (*heo*), or into a sacred stone. Of these two concepts it is evidently the *aunga* which corresponds most nearly with the concept of soul-substance. The stone statue on the burial-mound represents the deceased, and it is of great importance that it

[1] R. H. Codrington, *The Melanesians*, London, 1891, p. 249.
[2] C. E. Fox, *The Threshold of the Pacific*, 1925.

should be the *adaro*, corresponding with the ghost, which passes into it.

In the Banks Islands,[1] the soul is called *atai* in Mota and *talegi* in Motlav. It is believed to leave the body in vivid dreams and in fainting attacks, health depending on its presence and sound condition. A man can be deprived of his soul either by a ghost (*tamate*) or by a spirit (*vui*), or the soul may be merely damaged, the two events leading to illness of different degrees of severity. When the soul has been taken by a *vui*, it can be recovered by one called a *gismana*, who sends out his soul to seek the captured soul and restore it to its owner, this procedure corresponding closely with that of the Indonesian leeches.[2]

The *atai* of Mota is said to have signified originally something peculiarly connected with a person and sacred to him ; it might be a snake or a stone. We are told particularly that it does not mean a thing in which the soul is thought to be contained.[3] It is never used for the shadow, though the related *ata* is the word for the shadow in Samoa and for the reflected image in New Zealand.

In Maewo in the New Hebrides, the soul is called *tamaniu*, a word applied in Mota to the guardian animal, while in Pentecost Island and Lepers' Island the soul is *tamtegi*, a word related to the *tamate* which in other islands means ghost.

In Ambrim, the body is supposed to be tenanted by the *nin mauwan*, or spirit of life, which leaves the body temporarily in sleep and becomes the ghost (*temar*) at death. When an important man is seriously ill, the *nin mauwan* of his son or brother may leave his body in sleep and consult with the

---

[1] R. H. Codrington, *loc. cit.*
[2] W. H. R. Rivers, *Hist. Mel. Soc.*, vol. i, p. 165.
[3] R. H. Codrington and J. Palmer, *Mota Dictionary*, London, 1896, p. 7.

ghosts of the sick man's father or grandfather to learn the issue of the illness.

Pigs are believed to have a *nin mauwan*, but this does not become a *temar* or ghost when it dies. Nevertheless, the *nin mauwan* survives the death of the animal, and when a pig has been killed in certain ceremonies, its *nin mauwan* enters an image to await the coming of an ancestral ghost. It will be noted how close a parallel this presents with the belief of Florida that a pig has a *tarunga* but does not become a *tindalo*.

I will conclude my survey of Melanesian belief by referring to Fiji where we find in a definite form the twofold nature of the soul. T. Williams [1] tells us that some Fijians believe that man has two " spirits." One, the dark spirit, or shadow, goes to Hades, while the other, or light spirit, identified with the reflected image, stays near the place where a man dies. This belief resembles that of the Trobriands and San Cristoval, and if the information is to be trusted, it suggests that the dark spirit corresponds with the *aunga* of San Cristoval, and the light spirit with the shadow which enters a stone or stone image on the tomb.

With the exception of San Cristoval and Fiji, we have no definite evidence in Melanesia of the belief in two souls comparable with those of Indonesia and New Guinea. In most parts of Melanesia, the soul which leaves the body temporarily in sleep becomes the ghost, though here and there, as in Eddystone Island, we have evidence of a duality in the fate of the soul which may be a survival of a belief in its twofold nature.

Several of the properties attributed to the soul in Melanesia, such as its wanderings during sleep and its occasional embodiment in animal form, belong in Indonesia to the concept of

---

[1] *Fiji and the Fijians*, London, 1856, vol. i, p. 241. It must be noted that Fison failed to confirm this information and gives linguistic reasons to show that it is wrong. See Sir J. G. Frazer, *Taboo and the Perils of the Soul*, London, 1911, p. 92, n. 3.

soul-substance. Moreover, it will have been noted how frequently the survey just concluded has brought out the identification of the soul with the shadow. In New Guinea, this occurs in Tami and Kiriwina. In Melanesia, it is found in New Ireland, New Britain, Bougainville, the Shortland Islands, Eddystone Island, and San Cristoval, while the word for soul in Mota means shadow in Polynesia.

It is of great interest that in the two places of New Guinea and Melanesia which provide the clearest evidence of the duality of the soul, Kiriwina and San Cristoval, not only is there agreement in the identification of the soul with the shadow, but in both places the entity that is or becomes the ghost is identified with the reflection from water. In both places, it is the entity that corresponds the more closely with the soul-substance of Indonesia which is identified, as sometimes in Indonesia, with the shadow, while the entity that corresponds with the ghost of Indonesia is identified with the reflection from water. On the other hand, there is a very important difference between the two beliefs in that in the Trobriands it is the *baloma*, identified with the reflection, which goes to a distant home of the dead, while in San Cristoval it is the *aunga*, identified with the shadow, which passes to the distant Rodomana.

The identification of the shadow with the soul becomes particularly instructive when we trace out the vicissitudes which the Indonesian word for shadow has suffered in Melanesia. Among the Bahasa people and in Seran, the shadow is *nini, ninino, ninu, kaninu;* in Buru *nunin;* in north-east Celebes, *olinu*.[1] Among the Barriai of New Britain, the shadow is *anunu,* and it may be that the *nio* of the other end of the north coast of New Britain, which is used both for soul and shadow, is another form of the Indo-

---

[1] G. Friederici, *Wissenschaft. Ergebnisse,* iii. *Untersuchungen über eine Melanesische Wanderstrasse,* Berlin, 1913, p. 66. In some parts of Indonesia the banyan tree is called *nunu.*

nesian word. In the Shortland Islands, the word occurs more purely as *nunu*, used for both shadow and soul, and the relation to Indonesia is made clear by the accompanying use of the frequent Indonesian term for ghost, *nitu*, in these islands. *Nununa* occurs again in San Cristoval as the term for one of the two " souls " of the Bauro district.

In the Banks Islands and the New Hebrides, the Indonesian word again becomes obvious, though it is only in Ambrim that, in the form of *nin*, the word is used for the soul. In Mota, the shadow is *niniai*, while *nunuai* is used for a memory-image, such as the ringing of a sound in the ears. In Maewo in the New Hebrides, *nunu* is used for the relation between a person and the influence which affected his mother before his birth.[1] At Nogugu in Espiritu Santo, the shadow is *nunin* and in the island of Malo, *nunu*.

Nunu, or words evidently related to it, are thus used in many parts of Melanesia for the shadow, this being, so far as we know, the primary meaning of the word in Indonesia. In some parts of Melanesia, as in the Shortland Islands, San Cristoval, Ambrim, and probably in Duke of York Island, the word has also come to mean soul, while elsewhere it has acquired other meanings, all of which are related in some measure to the concept of soul.

It may be noted that if these ideas have passed from Indonesia to Melanesia and have become attached to the Melanesian concept of " soul," they are all derived from the more personal aspect of the soul-substance of Indonesia. We have no evidence from any part of Melanesia of the belief in the impersonal form of soul-substance which justifies this name. Sympathetic magic, spitting as a medical remedy, cannibalism, head-hunting and other customs which are explained in Indonesia by the presence of soul-substance are widely prevalent in Melanesia, but nowhere have we any hint

[1] See *History of Melanesian Society*, vol. i, p. 151.

H

that these customs rest on a belief in an essence permeating every part of man, animal or thing, by means of which its properties can be imparted to another being or object.

In one part of Melanesia, there is, however, an important set of beliefs which are possibly related to the Indonesian concept of soul-substance. In the Banks and Torres Islands, most of the religious and magical rites rest on the belief in a power or influence residing in the stones, leaves, words or other elements of the ritual. These objects are the vehicles by which an influence called *mana* is imparted from one being or object to another, just as an object which has been in contact with a person in Indonesia becomes a vehicle by which the spiritual influence called soul-substance within the person can be transmitted to another.

Behind this more or less impersonal application of the term *mana*, there is, as Codrington has pointed out,[1] a belief in a relation to a spiritual being, either a ghost or a spirit which has not been known to tenant a human form. If an object has *mana*, it is because it has been at some time associated with a person, human or spiritual, who was rich in *mana*. It is not generally known that this belief in a power, which, though derived from a person, is yet largely impersonal, has only a limited distribution in Melanesia and hardly occurs, at any rate under the term *mana*, outside the Banks and Torres Islands. In other parts of Melanesia, when the word *mana* occurs, it applies explicitly to the power of a personal being, human or spiritual, just as is the case in Polynesia. It would take me too far from my immediate topic to consider whether the Polynesian concept of *mana* may be related to the soul-substance of Indonesia. I must be content to point out that one special clue to the nature of Polynesian culture is the great development of sacred chieftainship which has taken place there. If immigrants became divine chiefs of the

---

[1] *The Melanesians*, p. 119.

people among whom they settled, and if these chiefs believed and taught that they were endowed with a special vital principle or essence, we have a basis for the process by which the soul-substance of Indonesia became the *mana* of Polynesia.[1]

In the Banks Islands, on the other hand, where sacred chieftainship has come to form part of the ritual of the ghost societies, it would seem as if the concept of soul-substance appears in a form more nearly like the Indonesian prototype, especially in its application to the purposes of religion and magic.

Having now concluded my survey of the various forms of belief in New Guinea and Melanesia which seem to be in any way related to the Indonesian concept of soul-substance, I may consider briefly whether it is possible to formulate any scheme to account for their relations.

The chief facts which need explanation are as follows. In Indonesia, there is a belief in an entity within a living man which is altogether distinct from the ghost which exists after death, this latter only coming into being at the moment of death as a kind of double of the deceased person. In New Guinea, there are beliefs so much like these that we can be confident that they are due to direct transmission either from Indonesia or from the source whence Indonesia itself obtained the beliefs in question. Such differences as there are would be due to the changes to be expected when abstract beliefs are transmitted to such lowly people as the Kai, or the natives of the mountainous districts visited by Mr Chinnery. It is noteworthy that, if one of Dr Malinowski's alternatives concerning the nature of the *baloma* be accepted, we have an almost exact reproduction of the Indonesian belief among the more advanced people of the Trobriand Islands.

When we pass from New Guinea eastwards, we find far

[1] Such a process would also explain the intense power of taboo claimed by Polynesian chiefs.

less kinship with the Indonesian point of view, and there is no evidence whatever for the belief in a soul-substance diffused throughout the body, although there are many customs which would be readily explained by such a concept. There is no obvious difference in intelligence between the natives of New Guinea and Melanesia—if anything, the Melanesians have the advantage in this respect—and if migrants from Indonesia succeeded in implanting their beliefs in the one place, it is difficult to see why there should have been so great a failure in the other.

A more important difference between the two regions is their distance from Indonesia. Once migrants from Indonesia have reached the shores of New Guinea, they are in contact with an island so large that it might almost be called a continent, the shores of which can be visited without calling upon the spirit of enterprise necessary for journeys to the more distant Solomon Islands. We can be fairly confident, therefore, that influences from Indonesia have permeated New Guinea but never reached Melanesia proper, and there is much in the cultures of the two regions to support this conjecture.

I suggest, therefore, that such evidence as we possess concerning the duality of the soul in Melanesia is due to some relatively early migration which reached both New Guinea and Melanesia, but has in the former place been overlaid by later influences from Indonesia which did not pass beyond New Guinea.

I have so far considered only the relation between the Indonesian concept and those of New Guinea and Melanesia. Mr Perry has given us good reason to suppose that the Indonesian concept was introduced into that region from the West. This raises the possibility that the cultural influence which brought the ideas in question to Indonesia travelled on to Melanesia, introducing there the idea of the duality of the soul. For reasons which I shall mention in a moment, it is of great importance that the district of Melanesia in which we have the most definite evidence of this duality is San Cristoval in the Solomon Islands. The Rev. C. E. Fox has recently[1] sent to Professor Elliot Smith and myself a record of the modes of burial of men of a certain chiefly clan in that and neighbouring islands. These funerary customs bear so close a resemblance to those of Egypt as to leave no reasonable doubt that travellers, imbued with the essential ideas of Egyptian culture, reached San Cristoval and introduced not only burial in pyramidal structures but also the custom of erecting a statue to serve as the residence of the ghost of the dead man. Such extraordinary resemblances between the mortuary customs of Egypt and San Cristoval justify us in comparing the beliefs concerning the soul held in the two places. I have already described the belief of San Cristoval. Of the two souls of that region, one leaves the body by the fontanelle or the mouth at death and sets out on a long journey to a distant place called Rodomana, while the other enters the statue upon the funeral mound. In Egypt there was also a belief in two souls, one of which flew to the sun in the form of a bird, while the other, called the *ka* or double, was believed to inhabit the statue representing the dead man erected within the *mastaba*. With the exception of the substitution of the journey to the vague Rodomana for the journey of the dead to the sun in Egypt, there is an almost exact resemblance between the beliefs of those two peoples, a resemblance far closer than that which exists between the beliefs of Egypt and Indonesia. The main fact, therefore, which has to be explained is the existence of the closest similarity of belief between the widely separated Egypt and San Cristoval, while between these two regions there is another set of beliefs common to Indonesia and New Guinea, having many points of resemblance with those of

---

[1] [This was written in 1919: the record has since been published as *The Threshold of the Pacific*, 1925.]

Egypt and San Cristoval, but of a more complex kind. This is the fact which calls for explanation, and for this purpose I venture to put forward the following hypothesis. Travellers imbued with the culture of Egypt, if not themselves Egyptian, reached Indonesia and passed on to Melanesia, the motive which lured them so far into the unknown being the desire for gold, pearls, and other precious objects, which has been shown by Mr Perry [1] to have furnished the motive for the early world-wide wanderings. In Melanesia, so distant from the main centres of the world's activity that it was rarely reached by outside influence, the Egyptian beliefs concerning the nature of the soul have been preserved with a high degree of faithful-ness. In Indonesia, on the other hand, so much nearer to the sources of modern civilization, the early belief has been over-laid by many later influences, and the idea originally introduced has been so modified as to produce the highly complex set of beliefs which are implied in the existing concept of soul-substance. Later movements have carried this modified and developed concept to New Guinea but have failed to reach Melanesia.

If further knowledge should support this hypothetical scheme, a remarkable consequence will follow, for which indeed we have already other evidence. This consequence is that if we wish to find ancient beliefs preserved with the greatest fidelity, we have to go to such distant and isolated spots as the islands of Melanesia, where the simple mentality of the people leads them to accept without any great modification beliefs which take their fancy, while the absence or scarcity of later external influence prevents the modification, or even oblitera-tion of beliefs, which are always liable to occur among more sophisticated peoples and in regions more open to the play of external influence. We are led to the extraordinary and at

---

[1] " The Relationship between the Geographical Distribution of Megalithic Monuments and Ancient Mines," *Mem. and Proc. Manchester Lit. and Phil. Soc.*, 1915.

first sight most improbable view that if we wish to obtain knowledge concerning the beliefs of the ancient world for which we have no literary evidence, we have to go, not to countries where the beliefs were held, nor to regions adjoining them which have been the seats of later civilizations, but to such distant and savage peoples as the natives of the Solomon Islands and the New Hebrides.

II

THE ETHNOLOGICAL ANALYSIS OF CULTURE [1]

DURING the last few years great additions have been made to our knowledge of the facts of anthropology—we have learnt much about different peoples scattered over the earth and we understand better how they act and think.   At the same time we have, I hope, made a very decided advance in our knowledge of the methods by means of which these facts are to be collected, so that they may rank in clearness and trustworthiness with the facts of other sciences.   When, however, we turn to the theoretical side of our subject, it is difficult to see any corresponding advance.   The main problems of the history of human society are little if at all nearer their solution, and there are even matters which a few years ago were regarded as settled which to-day are as uncertain as ever.   The reason for this is not far to seek ; it is that we have no general agreement about the fundamental principles upon which the theoretical work of our science is to be conducted.

In surveying the different schools of thought which guide theoretical work on human culture, a very striking fact at once presents itself.   In other and more advanced sciences, the guiding principles of the workers of different nations are the same.   The zoologists or botanists of France, Germany, America, our own and other countries are on common ground. They have in general the same principles and the same methods, and the work of all falls into a common scheme.

[1] Presidential Address to the Anthropological Section of the British Association for the Advancement of Science, Portsmouth, 1911.

Unfortunately this is not so in anthropology. At the present time there is so great a degree of divergence between the methods of work of the leading schools of different countries that any common scheme is impossible, and the members of one school wholly distrust the work of the others whose conclusions they believe to be founded on a radically unsound basis.

I propose to consider in this address one of the most striking of these divergences, but, before doing so, I will put as briefly as possible what seem to me to be the chief characters of the leading schools of different countries. I will begin with that dominant among ourselves. The theoretical anthropology of this country is inspired primarily by the idea of evolution founded on a psychology common to mankind as a whole, and, further, a psychology differing in no way from that of civilized man. The efforts of British anthropologists are devoted to tracing out the evolution of custom and institution. Where similarities are found in different parts of the world, it is assumed, almost as an axiom, that they are due to independent origin and development, and this in its turn is ascribed to the fundamental similarity of the workings of the human mind all over the world, so that, given similar conditions, similar customs and institutions will come into existence and develop on the same lines.

In France, as among ourselves, we find that the chief interest is in evolution, and the difference is in the principles upon which this evolution is to be studied. It is to the psychological basis of the work of British anthropologists that objection is chiefly made. It is held that the psychology of the individual cannot be used as a guide to the collective actions of men in early stages of social evolution, still less the psychology of the individual whose social ideas have been moulded by the long ages of evolution which have made our own society what it is. It is urged that the study of sociology requires the application of principles and methods of investigation peculiar to itself.[1]

About America it is less easy to speak, because it is unusual in that country to deal to any great extent with general theoretical problems. The anthropologists of America are so fully engaged in the attempt to record what is left of the ancient cultures of their own country that they devote little attention to those general questions to which we, with no ancient culture at our doors, devote so much attention. There seems, however, to be a distinct movement in progress in America which puts the evolutionary point of view on one side and is inclined to study social problems from the purely psychological point of view, the psychological standpoint, however, approaching that of the British school more nearly than that of the French.[2]

It is when we come to Germany that we find the most fundamental difference in standpoint and method. It is true that in Adolf Bastian Germany produced a scholar thoroughly familiar with the evolutionary standpoint, and the *Elementargedanke* of that worker forms a most convenient expression for the psychological means whereby evolution is supposed to have proceeded. In recent years, however, there has been a very decided movement opposed to Bastian and the whole evolutionary school. In some cases this has formed part of that general revolt so prominent in Germany, not merely against Darwinism, but it seems even against the whole idea of evolution. In other cases, the objection is less fundamental, and has been not so much to the idea of evolution itself as to

---

[1] I refer here especially to the work of the " sociological " school of Durkheim and his followers. For an account of their principles and methods see *L'Année sociologique*, which began to appear in 1898 ; Durkheim, *Les Règles de la Méthode Sociologique*, Paris ; and Lévy-Bruhl, *Les fonctions mentales dans les sociétés inférieures*, Paris, 1910.

[2] See especially A. L. Kroeber, " Classificatory Systems of Relationship," *Journ. Roy. Anthr. Inst.*, 1919, xxxix, 77 ; and Goldenweiser, " Totemism : An Analytical Study," *Journ. Amer. Folk-Lore*, 1910, xxiii.

the lines upon which it has been customary to study this evolution.

This movement, which by those who follow it is called the geographical movement, but which, I think, may be more fitly styled ' ethnological,' was originated by Ratzel, who was first led definitely in this direction by a study of the armour made of rods or plates or laths which is found in North America, northern Asia, including Japan, and in a less developed form in some of the islands of the Pacific Ocean.[1] Ratzel believed that the resemblances he found could only be explained by direct transmission from one people to another and was led by further study to become an untiring opponent of the *Elementargedanke* of Bastian and of the idea of independent evolution based on a community of thought.[2] He has even suggested that the idea of independent origin is the anthropological equivalent of the spontaneous generation of the biologist and that anthropology is now going through a phase of development from which biology has long emerged.

The movement initiated by Ratzel has made great progress, especially through the work of Graebner [3] and of P. W. Schmidt.[4] It has resulted in an important series of works in which the whole field of anthropological research is approached in a manner wholly different from that customary

---

[1] *Sitzber. d. Akad. d. Wiss. München*, Hist. Cl., 1886, p. 181.
[2] See especially *Anthropogeographie*, 1891, Th. ii, 705, and " Die geographische Methode in der Ethnographie," *Geograph. Zeitsch.*, 1897, iii, 268.
[3] See especially Graebner, *Methode der Ethnologie*, Heidelberg, 1911, and " Die melanesische Bogenkultur und ihre Verwandten," *Anthropos*, 1909, iv, 726. The annual *Ethnologica*, edited by W. Foy, is devoted to the illustration of this school of thought.
[4] See especially " L'Origine de l'Idée de Dieu," *Anthropos*, iii-v, 1908-10, and " Grundlinien einer Vergleichung der Religion u. Mythologie der austronesischen Völker, *Denksch. d. Akad. d. Wiss. Wien*, Phil.-hist. Kl., 1910, liii. Schmidt differs from Graebner in limiting the application of the ethnological method to regions with general affinities of culture. Otherwise he remains an adherent of the doctrine of independent origin. (See " Panbabylonismus und ethnologischer Elementargedanke," *Mitt. d. anthrop. Gesellsch. in Wien*, 1908, xxxviii, 73.)

in this country.[1]   I must content myself with one example to illustrate the difference of standpoint which separates the two schools.   Few subjects have attracted more interest in this and other countries than the study of primitive decoration. In the decorative art of all lands there are found transitions from designs representing the human form or those of animals and plants to purely geometrical patterns.   In this country it has been held, I think I may say universally, that in these transitions we have evidence for an evolutionary process which in all parts of the world has led mankind to what may be called the degradation and conventionalization of human, animal or plant designs, so that in course of time they become mere geometrical forms.

To the modern German school, on the other hand, these transitions are examples of the blending of two cultures, one possessing the practice of decorating their objects with human, animal or plant designs, while the art of the other is based on the use of geometrical forms.   The transitions which have been taken to be evidence of independent processes of evolution based on psychological tendencies common to mankind are by the modern German school ascribed to the mixture of cultures and of peoples.   Further, similar patterns, even one so simple as the spiral, when found in widely separated regions of the earth, are held to have been due to the influence of one and the same culture.

I have chosen this example because it illustrates the immense divergence in thought and method between the two schools, but the difference runs through the whole range of the subject.   In every case where British anthropologists see evolution, either in the forms of material objects or in social

---

[1] It must not be understood from this account that all German anthropologists are adherents of the ethnological school.   There are still those who follow the doctrines of Bastian, which have undergone an interesting modification through the adoption of the biological principle of Convergence (see p. 141).

and religious institutions, the modern German school sees only the evidence of mixture of cultures, either with or without an accompanying mixture of the races to which these cultures belonged.

It will, I think, be evident that this difference of attitude between British and German workers is one of fundamental and vital importance. When we find the chief workers of two nations thus approaching their subject from two radically different, and it would seem, incompatible standpoints, it is evident that there must be something very wrong.

The situation is one which has an especial interest for me in that I have been led quite independently to much the same general position as that of the German school by the results of my own work in Oceania with the Percy Sladen Trust Expedition. With no knowledge of the work of this school, I was led by my facts to see how much, in the past, I had myself ignored considerations arising from racial mixture and the blending of cultures, and I will briefly sketch the history of my own conversion.

Much of my time in Oceania was devoted to survey work, in which I collected especially the systems of relationship of every place I visited, together with other facts concerning social organization I was able to gather. I began my theoretical study by a comparison of the various forms of these systems of relationship, disregarding at first the linguistic nature of the terms. From the study of these systems, I was able to demonstrate the existence either in the present or the past of a number of extraordinary and anomalous forms of marriage, such as marriage with the daughter's daughter and with the wife of the father's father,[1] all of which become explicable if there once existed widely throughout Melanesia a state which is known as the dual organization of society with matrilineal descent and accompanied by a condition of

---

[1] These terms are used in the classificatory sense.

dominance of the old men which enabled them to monopolize all the young women of the community. Taking this as my starting-point, I was then able to trace out a consistent and definite scheme of the history of marriage in Melanesia from a condition in which persons normally and naturally married certain relatives, to one in which wives are purchased with whom no relationship whatever can be traced, and I was able to fit many other features of the social structure of Melanesia into this scheme. So far my work was of a purely evolutionary character, and only served to strengthen me in my previous standpoint.

I then turned my attention to the linguistic side of the systems of relationship, and a study of the terms themselves showed that these fell into two main classes : one class generally diffused throughout Oceania, while the terms of the other class differed very considerably in different cultural regions. Further, it became clear that the terms of the first class denoted relationships which my comparative study of the forms of the systems had shown to have suffered change, while the terms which varied greatly in different parts of Oceania denoted relationships, such as those of the mother and mother's brother, which there was no reason to believe had suffered any great change in status. From these facts I inferred that, at the time of the most primitive stage of Melanesian society of which I had evidence, there had been great linguistic diversity which had been transformed into the relative uniformity now found in Melanesia by the incoming of a people from without, through whose influence the change I had traced had taken place, and from whose language the generally diffused terms of relationship had been borrowed. It was through the combined study of social forms and of language that I was led to see that the change I had traced was not a spontaneous evolution, but one which had taken place under the influence of the blending of peoples. The combined morphological and linguistic study of systems of relationship had led me to recognize that a definite course of social development had taken place in an aboriginal society under the influence of an immigrant people.

I turned next to a Melanesian institution, that of secret societies, concerning which I had been able to gather much new material, and it soon became probable that these societies properly belonged neither to the aboriginal culture nor to that of the immigrants, but had arisen as the result of the interaction of the two ; that, in fact, these secret societies had had their source in the need felt by the immigrants for the secret practice of the rites they had brought with them from their former home. A comparison of the ritual of the secret societies with the institutions of other parts of Oceania then made it appear that the main features of the culture of these immigrants had been patrilineal descent, or at any rate definite recognition of the relation between father and child, a cult of the dead, the institution of taboo, and, lastly, certain relations with animals and plants which were probably allied to totemism, if they were not totemism itself in a fully developed form.

Further study made it clear that those I have called the immigrant people, though possessing these features in common, had reached Melanesia at different times and with several decided differences of culture, but that probably there had been two main streams : one which peopled Polynesia and became widely diffused throughout Melanesia, which was characterized by the use of kava ; another which came later and penetrated much less widely, that brought with it the practice of chewing betel-mixture. Traces of a third stream, the earliest of all, are probably to be found here and there throughout Melanesia, while still another element is provided by recent Polynesian influence. It became evident that the present condition of Melanesian society has come into being through the blending of an aboriginal population with various peoples from without, and it therefore became necessary to ascertain to which of the cultures possessed by these peoples the present-day customs and institutions of Melanesia belong, always keeping in mind the possibility that some of these institutions may not have belonged to any one of the cultures, but may have arisen as the result of the interaction of two or more of the blending peoples.

I must be content with this brief sketch of my scheme of the history of Melanesian society, for my object is to point out that if Melanesian society possesses the complexity and the heterogeneity of character I have indicated, and is the resultant of the mixture of three or four main cultures, it cannot be right to take out of the complex any institution or belief and regard it as primitive merely because Melanesian culture on the whole is more or less primitive. It is probable that some of the immigrants into Melanesia had a relatively advanced culture, possibly even that the institutions and ideas they brought with them had been taken from a culture higher still, and, therefore, when we bring forward any Melanesian institution or belief as an example of primitive thinking or acting, our first duty should be to inquire to which stratum of Melanesian culture it belongs.

Here is an example to illustrate my meaning. No concept of Melanesian culture has bulked more largely in recent speculation than that of *mana*, the mysterious virtue to which the magico-religious rites of Melanesia are believed to owe their efficacy. This word now seems on its way to enter the English language as a term for that power or virtue which induces the emotions of awe and wonder, and thus not only provides a most important element in the specific mental states which underlie religion, but also plays much the same part in the early history of magic. In recent speculation, the idea of *mana* is coming to be regarded as the basis of religious ideas and practices preceding the animism which, following Professor Tylor, we have for long regarded as the earliest form of religion. *Mana* is thus held to be not only the foundation of pre-animistic religion, but also the basis of that primitive element of human culture which can hardly be called either religion or magic, but is the common source from which both have been derived. If I am right in my analysis of Oceanic culture, the Melanesian concept of *mana* is not a suitable basis for these speculations. It is certain that the word *mana* belongs to the culture of the immigrants into Melanesia and not to that of the aborigines. It is, of course, possible that, though the word belongs to the immigrant culture, the ideas which it connotes may belong to a more primitive stratum, but this is a pure assumption and one which I believe to be contrary to all probability. At any rate, we can be confident that even if the ideas connoted by the term *mana* belong to or were shared by the primitive stratum of Melanesian society, they must have been largely modified by the influence of the alien but superior culture from which the word itself has been taken. I believe that the Melanesian evidence can legitimately be used in favour of the view that the power or virtue denoted by *mana* is a fundamental element of religion. The analysis of culture, however, indicates that it is not legitimate to use the Melanesian evidence to support the primitiveness of the concept of *mana*. This evidence certainly does not support the view that the concept of *mana* is more primitive than animism, for the immigrants were already in a very advanced stage of animistic religion, a cult of the dead being certainly one of the most definite of their religious institutions.

Further, I believe that the use of the term *mana* in Melanesia in connection with magic, as a term for that attribute of objects used in magic to which they owe their efficacy, is due to an extension of the original meaning of the term, and that

I

it would only be misleading to use the Melanesian facts as evidence in favour of the concept of *mana* as underlying primitive magic. Here, again, I do not wish to deny that a concept such as that denoted by *mana* may be a primitive element of magic; all that I wish to point out is that the Melanesian evidence cannot properly be used to support this view, for the use of the term in connection with magic in Melanesia is not primitive but secondary and relatively late.

The point, then, on which I wish to insist is that, if cultures are complex, their analysis is a preliminary step which is necessary if speculations concerning the evolution of human society, its beliefs and practices, are to rest on a firm foundation.

I have so far dealt only with Melanesia. It is obvious that the same principle, that analysis of culture must precede speculations concerning the evolution of institutions, is of wider application, but I have space only to deal, and that very briefly, with one other region.

No part of the world has attracted more attention in recent anthropological speculation than Australia, and at the bottom of these speculations, at any rate in this country, there has usually been the idea, openly expressed or implicitly understood, that, in the culture of this region, we have a homogeneous example of primitive human society. From the time that I first became acquainted with Australian sociology, I have wondered at the complacency with which certain features of Australian social organization have been regarded, and especially the combination of the dual organization and matrimonial classes with what appear to be totemic clans like those of other parts of the world. This co-existence of two different forms of social organization side by side has seemed to me the fundamental problem of Australian society, and I confess that till lately, obsessed as I see now I have been by a crude evolutionary point of view, the condition' has seemed an absolute mystery.[1] A comparison, however, of Australia and Melanesia has now led me to see that probably we have in Australia not merely another example of mixture of cultures, but even another resultant of mixture of the same or closely similar components as those which have peopled Melanesia : viz., a mixture of a people possessing the dual organization and matrilineal descent with one organized in totemic clans, possessing either patrilineal descent, or at any rate clear recognition of the relation between father and child. This is no new view, having been already advanced, though in a different form, by Graebner [2] and P. W. Schmidt.[3] If further research should show Australian society to possess such complexity, it will at once become obvious that here also ethnological analysis must precede any theoretical use of the facts of Australian society in support of evolutionary speculations.

It may be objected that we all recognize the complexity of culture, and indeed in the study of regions such as the Mediterranean, where we possess historical evidence, it is this complexity which forms the chief subject of discussion. Further, where we possess historical evidence, as in the cases of the Hindu and Mahommedan invasions into the Malay Archipelago, all anthropologists are fully alive to the complexities and difficulties introduced thereby into the study of culture ; but where we have no such historical evidence, the complexity of culture is almost wholly ignored by those who use these cultures in their attempts to demonstrate the origin and course of development of human institutions.

I have now reached the first stage of my argument. I have tried to indicate that evolutionary speculations can have no

---

[1] I may note here that Mr Lang, after having considered this problem from the purely " evolutionary " standpoint (*Anthropological Essays presented to E. B. Tylor*, p. 203), concludes with the words, " We seem lost in a wilderness of difficulties."

[2] *Zeitsch. f. Ethnol.*, 1905, xxxvii, 28, and " Zur australischen Religionsgeschichte," *Globus*, 1909, xcvi, 341.

[3] See especially *Zeitsch. f. Ethnol.*, 1909, xli, 340.

firm basis unless there has been a preceding analysis of the cultures and civilizations now spread over the earth's surface. Without such analysis it is impossible to say whether an institution or belief possessed by a people who seem simple and primitive may not really be the product of a relatively advanced culture forming but one element of a complexity which at first sight seems simple and homogeneous.

Before proceeding further, I should like to guard against a possible misconception. Some of those who are interested in the ethnological analysis of culture regard it not only as the first but as the only task of the anthropology of to-day. I cannot too strongly express my disagreement with this view. Because I have insisted on the importance of ethnological analysis, that does not imply that I underrate the need for the psychological study of customs and institutions. If the necessity for the ethnological analysis of culture be recognized, this psychological study becomes more complicated and difficult than it has seemed to be in the past, but that makes it none the less essential. Side by side with ethnological analysis, there must go the attempt to fathom the modes of thought of different peoples, to understand their ways of regarding and classifying the facts of the universe. It is only by the combination of ethnological and psychological analysis that we shall make any real advance.

Having shown the importance of ethnological analysis, I now propose to consider the process of analysis itself and the principles on which it should and must be based, if it is in its turn to have any firm foundation. In the analysis of any culture, a difficulty which soon meets the investigator is that he has to determine what is due to mere contact and what is due to intimate intermixture, such intermixture, for instance, as is produced by the permanent blending of one people with another either through warlike invasion or peaceful settlement. The fundamental weakness of most of the attempts hitherto made to analyse existing cultures is that they have had their starting-point in the study of material objects, and the reason for this is obvious. Owing to the fact that material objects can be collected by anyone and subjected at leisure to prolonged study by experts, our knowledge of the distribution of material objects and of the technique of their manufacture has very far outrun that of the less material elements. What I wish now to point out is that in distinguishing between the effects of mere contact and the intermixture of peoples, material objects are the least trustworthy of all the constituents of culture. Thus, in Melanesia we have the clearest evidence that material objects and processes can spread by mere contact without any true admixture of peoples and without influence on other features of the culture. While the distribution of material objects is of the utmost importance in suggesting at the outset community of culture, and while it is of equal importance in the final process of determining points of contact and in filling in the details of the mixture of cultures, it is the least satisfactory guide to the actual blending of peoples, which must form the solid foundation of the ethnological analysis of culture. The case for the value of magico-religious institutions is not much stronger. Here, again, in Melanesia there is little doubt that whole cults can pass from one people to another without any real intermixture of peoples. I do not wish to imply that such religious institutions can pass from people to people with the ease of material objects, but to point out that there is evidence that they can and do so pass with very little, if any, admixture of peoples or of the deeper and more fundamental elements of the culture. Much more important is language, and if you will think over the actual conditions when one people either visit or settle among another, this greater importance will be obvious. Let us imagine a party of Melanesians visiting a Polynesian island, staying there for a few weeks and then returning home (and here I am not taking a fictitious occurrence but one which really happens). We can readily understand that the visitors may take with them their betel mixture and thereby introduce the custom of betel-chewing into a new home ; we can readily understand that they may introduce an ornament to be worn in the nose and another to be worn on the chest ; that tales that they tell will be remembered, and dances they perform will be imitated. A few Melanesian words may pass into the language of the Polynesian island, especially as names for the objects or processes which the strangers have introduced, but it is incredible that the strangers should thus in a short visit produce any extensive change in the vocabulary and still more that they should modify the structure of the language. Such changes can never be the result of mere contact or transient settlement, but must always indicate a far more deeply-seated and fundamental process of blending of peoples and cultures.

Few will perhaps hesitate to accept this position, but I expect my next proposition to meet with more scepticism, and yet I believe it to be widely, though not universally, true.[1] This proposition is that the social structure, the framework of society, is still more fundamentally important and still less easily changed except as the result of the intimate blending of peoples, and for that reason furnishes by far the firmest foundation on which to base the process of analysis of culture. I cannot hope to establish the truth of this proposition in the course of a brief chapter, and I propose to consider one line of evidence only.

At the present moment we have before our eyes an object-lesson in the spread of our own people over the earth's surface, and we are thus able to study how external influence affects different elements of culture. What we find is that mere

---

[1] There are definite exceptions in Melanesia ; places where the social structure has been transformed, though the ancient language persists.

contact is able to transmit much in the way of material culture. A passing vessel which does not even anchor may be able to transmit iron, while European weapons may be used by people who have never even seen a white man. Again, missionaries introduce the Christian religion among people who cannot speak a word of English or any language but their own, or only use such European words as have been found necessary to express ideas or objects connected with the new religion. There is evidence how readily language may be affected, and here again the present day suggests a mechanism by which such a change takes place. English is now becoming the language of the Pacific and of other parts of the world, through its use as a *lingua franca*, which enables natives who speak different languages to converse not only with Europeans, but with one another, and I believe that this has often been the mechanism in the past ; that, for instance, the introduction of what we now call the Melanesian structure of language was due to the fact that the language of the immigrant people who settled in a region of great linguistic diversity came to be used as a *lingua franca*, and thus gradually became the basis of the languages of the whole people.

But now let us turn to social structure. We find in Oceania islands where Europeans have been settled as missionaries or traders perhaps for fifty or a hundred years ; we find the people wearing European clothes and European ornaments, using European utensils, and even European weapons when they fight ; we find them holding the beliefs and practising the ritual of a European religion ; we find them speaking a European language often even among themselves, and yet investigation shows that much of their social structure remains thoroughly native and uninfluenced not only in its general form, but often even in its minute details. The external influence has swept away the whole material culture, so that objects of native origin are manufactured only to sell to tourists ;

it has substituted a wholly new religion and destroyed every
material, if not every moral, vestige of the old ; it has caused
great modification and degeneration of the old language ;
and yet it may have left the social structure in the main untouched. And the reasons for this are clear. Most of the
essential social structure of a people lies below the surface ;
it is so literally the foundation of the whole life of the people
that it is not seen ; it is not obvious, but can only be reached
by patient and laborious exploration.   I will give a few specific
instances. In several islands of the Pacific, some of which
have had European settlers on them for more than a century,
a most important position in the community is occupied by
the father's sister.[1]   If any native of these islands were asked
who is the most important person in the determination of his
life-history, he would answer, " My father's sister," and yet
the place of this relative in the social structure has remained
absolutely unrecorded, and, I believe, absolutely unknown to
the European settlers in these islands. Again, Europeans
have settled in Fiji for more than a century, and yet it was
only during this summer [2] that I heard from Mr A. M. Hocart,
who was working there, that there is the clearest evidence of
what is known as the dual organization of society as a working
social institution at the present time.   How unobtrusive such
a fundamental fact of social structure may be comes home to
me in this case very strongly, for it wholly eluded my own
observation during a visit three years ago.

     Lastly, the most striking example of the permanence of
social structure which I have met is in the Hawaiian Islands.
There the original native culture is reduced to the merest
wreckage.   So far as material objects are concerned, the people
are like ourselves ; the old religion has gone, though there
probably still persists some of the ancient magic.   The people
themselves have so dwindled in number, and the political

----

[1] See *Folk-Lore*, 1910, xxi, 42.   [2] 1911.

conditions are so altered, that the social structure has also necessarily been greatly modified. Yet I was able to ascertain that one of its elements, an element which I believe to form the deepest layer of the foundation, the very bed-rock of social structure, the system of relationship, is still in use un-changed. I was able to obtain a full account of the system as actually used at the present time, and found it to be exactly the same as that recorded forty years ago by Morgan and Hyde, and I obtained evidence that the system is still deeply interwoven with the intimate mental life of the people.

If, then, social structure has this fundamental and deeply seated character, if it is the least easily changed and only changed as the result either of actual blending of peoples or of the most profound political changes, the obvious inference is that it is with social structure that we must begin the attempt to analyse culture and to ascertain how far community of culture is due to the blending of peoples, how far to trans-mission through mere contact or transient settlement.

The considerations I have brought forward have, however, in my opinion, an importance still more fundamental. If social institutions have this relatively great degree of perman-ence, if they are so deeply seated and so closely interwoven with the deepest instincts and sentiments of a people that they can only gradually suffer change, will not the study of this change give us our surest criterion of what is early and what is late in any given culture, and thereby furnish a guide for the analysis of culture ? Such criteria of early and late are necessary if we are to arrange the cultural elements reached by our analysis in order of time, and it is very doubtful whether mere geographical distribution itself will ever furnish a sufficient basis for this purpose. I may remind you here that before the importance of the complexity of Melanesian culture had forced itself on my mind, I had already succeeded in tracing out a course for the development of the structure of

Melanesian society, and after the complexity of the culture had been established, I did not find it necessary to alter anything of essential importance in this scheme. I suggest, therefore, that while the ethnological analysis of cultures must furnish a necessary preliminary to any general evolutionary speculations, there is one element of culture which has so relatively high a degree of permanence that its course of development may furnish a guide to the order in time of the different elements into which it is possible to analyse a given complex.

If the development of social structure is thus to be taken as a guide to assist the process of analysis, it is evident that there will be involved a logical process of considerable complexity in which there will be the danger of arguing in a circle. If, however, the analysis of culture is to be the primary task of the anthropologist, it is evident that the logical methods of the science will attain a complexity far exceeding those hitherto in vogue. I believe that the only logical process which will in general be found possible will be the formulation of hypothetical working schemes into which the facts can be fitted, and that the test of such schemes will be their capacity to fit in with themselves, or, as we generally express it, "explain" new facts as they come to our knowledge. This is the method of other sciences which deal with conditions as complex as those of human society. In many other sciences, these new facts are discovered by experiment. In our science, they must be found by exploration, not only of the cultures still existent in living form, but also of the buried cultures of past ages.

And here is the hopeful aspect of our subject. I believe our present store of facts, at any rate on the less material sides of culture, to form but a very small part of that which is yet to be obtained, and will be obtained unless we very wilfully neglect our opportunities. There is a vast body of knowledge waiting to be collected by means of which to test the truth of schemes of the history of mankind, not only of his migrations and settlements, but of the institutions and objects which have arisen at different stages of this history and developed into various forms throughout the world.

And this brings me to my concluding topic. I have tried to show that any speculations concerning the history of human institutions can only have a sound basis if cultures have first been analysed into their component elements, but I do not wish for one moment to depreciate the importance of attempts to seek for the origin and early history of human institutions. To me the analysis of culture is merely the means to an end which would have little interest if it did not show us the way to the proper understanding of the history of human institutions. The importance of the facts of ethnology in the study of civilized culture is now generally recognized. You can hardly take up a modern work dealing with any aspect of human thought and activity without finding reference to the customs and institutions of savage or barbarous peoples. It is becoming recognized that a study of these helps us to understand much that is obscure in our own institutions or in those of other great civilizations of the present or the past. Further, there can be no doubt that we are only at the threshold of a new movement in learning which is being opened by this comparative study.

It is a cruel irony that just as the importance of the facts and conclusions of ethnological research is thus becoming recognized, and just as we are beginning to learn sound principles and methods for use both in the field and in the study, the material of our science is vanishing. Not only is the march of our own civilization into the hitherto undisturbed places of the earth more rapid than it has ever been before, but this advance has made more easy the spread of other destroying agencies. In many parts of such a region as Melanesia, it is even now only from the old men that any trustworthy information can be obtained, and it is no exaggeration to say that with the death of every old man there and in many other places there goes, and goes for ever, knowledge the disappearance of which the scholars of the future will regret as the scholars of the past regretted such an event as the disappearance of the library of Alexandria. There is no other science which is in quite the same position. The nervous system of an animal, the metabolism of a plant, the condition of the South Pole, for instance, will in a hundred or even a thousand years hence, be essentially what they are to-day, but long before the shorter of those times has passed, most, if not all, of the lower cultures now found on different parts of the earth will have wholly disappeared or have suffered such change that little will be learnt from them. Fortunately, the need for ethnographical research is now forcing itself on the attention of those who have to deal with savage or barbarous peoples. Statesmen have begun to recognize the practical importance of knowing the institutions of those they have to govern, and missionary societies are beginning to see, what every wise missionary has long known, that it is necessary to understand the ideas and customs of those whose lives they are trying to reform. Still, we must not be content with these more or less official movements. There is ample scope, indeed urgent need, for individual effort and for non-official enterprise. It is not all who can go into the field and do the needed work themselves, but there are none who cannot in some way help to promote ethnographical research. We have before us one of those critical occasions which must be seized at once if they are to be seized at all : the occasion of a need which to future generations will seem to have been so obvious that its neglect will be held an enduring reproach to the science of our time.

B.—CULTURAL AND HISTORICAL

I

CONVERGENCE IN HUMAN CULTURE

THE comparative study of human societies has shown the presence of striking resemblances between peoples widely separated from one another in space, physical character and culture. These resemblances are often superficial, and close examination may show that customs, apparently identical, really have a very different nature. Nevertheless, even when the utmost allowance is made in this direction, there remains a vast number of resemblances, not merely in general character but often in minute detail, which it is the business of the science of ethnology to explain.

The theories which have been put forward to account for these resemblances are of two main kinds. According to one kind, they depend upon the direct transmission of customs or institutions from one place to another by the wanderings of peoples. According to the other, they have arisen independently in a process of " evolution " owing to the similarity of the workings of the human mind when exposed to similar conditions. These two main lines of explanation may be called respectively the theories of Transmission and of Independent Origin.

Theories of independent origin again fall into two groups : those in which the similarities are conceived as being the final outcome of two parallel lines of development, and those in which the similar customs have arisen out of dissimilar customs or institutions through the influence of similar external conditions, in which parallel or divergent lines of development have converged so as to produce customs similar to one another. These two modes of explanation may be spoken of respectively as parallelism and convergence.

By German ethnologists, following Adolf Bastian, two varieties of parallelism are recognized ; those in which the similarity depends on the presence of some mental character common to the whole of Mankind, the *Elementargedanke* of Bastian ; the other, in which the similarity depends on the common presence of a mental factor which is not universally present among mankind, but is the peculiar possession of one people, the *Völkergedanke* of Bastian.

The process of convergence which is the special subject of this chapter corresponds with the process similarly named in biology. Hence the term " convergence " is used for such cases as the resemblance in character between fishes and marine mammals. Here members of two divisions of the animal kingdom, which in the process of evolution have diverged widely from one another, have again converged in certain respects as the result of adaptation to aquatic life. Another example of a different kind is the resemblance between animals of very different kinds which may be produced by those conditions we call Mimicry. The object of this chapter is to inquire how far it is possible to use a similar process of convergence in ethnology, and how far it helps us to understand the similarities of human custom in different parts of the world.

It will be useful to begin by considering more exactly what the concept of convergence means to the biologist. The similarity between the whale and the fish, far removed from one another in their most essential characters, is conceived as having been due to a process of adaptation carried on through many generations, in which the fundamental differences between the two animals have been covered, more or less superficially, by a number of resemblances. In most cases the biologist has to be content with the position that the changes which have occurred in one or other of the two convergent lines of development have been brought about by external forces, and it is only exceptionally that he is able to formulate any exact scheme of the process by which the changes have been brought about.   Even if able to formulate the functional and structural changes by which the mammal has responded to aquatic conditions, he is still left with the unsolved mystery of the process by which such changes have been transmitted from generation to generation.   Convergence, to the zoologist, too often remains little more than a convenient term for a process he does not understand.

Owing to its modernity, human society furnishes a more promising field than do many closely-allied varieties of mankind ; the persistence of peoples who more or less closely represent stages of his progress and intermediate links in his development are probably far more numerous; the less rigorous conditions of man's development have not so far had so destructive an effect on the intermediate products.   Thus, there is far more hope of tracing out the process by which the convergence has taken place than there is in zoology.   The ethnologist has no right to be content, even in the present imperfect state of our knowledge, with convergence as an unanalysed concept ; it is possible even now to formulate the various conditions which can be included under this comprehensive term, and inquire whether it is possible to formulate a theory, or theories, of the process which will be useful as guides and stimuli to research.

I will first consider the processes which underlie convergence, regarded solely as a mode of independent origin.

It is agreed that the term convergence shall be used for a process whereby dissimilar social conditions resemble one another.   The problem to be studied is the mechanism by which this convergence is produced.   Two courses are possible :

one to inquire into the mental states which act as motives for the convergent customs ; the other, is to seek out the historical antecedents of the convergent customs, and to trace out as far as possible the changes by which the convergence has been brought about. Let us consider these two alternatives and take the custom of head-hunting as an illustration.

If we inquire into the motives which not only may have produced the practice of head-hunting but do as a matter of fact actuate it at the present time, we find that one is the desire to preserve a memento of a meritorious feat. In a word, the idea underlying head-hunting may be that the head is regarded as a trophy. In our own culture, both of the present and the past, the appeal of the trophy to the human mind is very great. One can hardly enter a house in any part of the world without seeing signs of this love of trophies. The place of the turtle-shell of our kitchens is taken by the pig's jaw-bone or the fish's head, and the captured guns of our wars find their substitutes in the scalp, skull or jaw of a slaughtered enemy. It may be supposed that the taking of heads is merely an example of the love of trophies which appears to be a universal characteristic of mankind. Merely from this point of view head-hunting would provide examples of the *Elementargedanke* of Bastian, and whether we call it parallelism or convergence would depend on whether it had arisen in similar or dissimilar societies.

There still remains, however, the question why it should be the head which is thus taken and preserved ; this question must be answered if our explanation is to be complete. It is not enough to say that the head is the natural trophy, for we find peoples who use ears or hands for this purpose. If we examine the cultures in which head-hunting flourishes, and I will take as examples the peoples of the Malay Archipelago, Melanesia, and America, we find the idea that the head is the representative of the body widespread among them. In Melanesia and Polynesia, for instance, the sanctity of sacred persons, such as chiefs, is centred in the head. It is especially the head which may not be touched ; it is the head on which the shadow of another person must not fall ; it is the head which is used as the sign or symbol of another individual. It is evident that among these peoples the rôle of the head as the representative of the body is not merely a floating idea liable to influence the practices of a people now and then or here and there, but it is an idea which has become the centre of an organized system of social practices. Though the idea in some more or less vague form may be present universally among mankind, it is only among certain peoples that it has acquired that definite character which makes it the psychological basis of groups of social processes. So far as we know, this importance of the head as a prominent element in social custom is especially pronounced in Austronesian culture, and if it were found to be peculiar to these peoples, we might regard it as a type of the *Völkergedanke* of Bastian. But we should still be left with the problem as to why this group of peoples have come to possess the idea in so potent and special a form. From the psychological point of view, there is no hope of further progress ; it is necessary to inquire into the general social conditions with which the practice of head-hunting is associated.

Let us first ask what is done with the heads when they are taken. If they are merely hung in the dwelling-house or club, we can be provisionally content to regard them as trophies, but if they are found to enter into the social and religious life of the people, we can not be so content.

In Indonesia and Melanesia, heads are used in rites connected with such essential crafts as house-building and canoe-making. In the head-hunting districts of Melanesia, no house could be inhabited, no canoe be launched if heads were not at

K

hand to be used as the offering which forms part of an organized cult of the dead. The motive for head-hunting in these regions is not that of glory or the revival of memories of success, but depends on a religious need so great that many of the chief acts of life cannot be properly performed without it. If in some places head-hunting is thus closely connected with an ancestor-cult, the possibility arises that it may be so elsewhere, and that the use of heads as trophies which appears to us to be a sufficient motive may only be a survival of a former dependence on social and religious needs of the same kind as those which underlie the practice in Melanesia and Indonesia.

If now we examine the head-hunting of America, we find undoubted indications of a connection with a cult of the dead, suggesting that here also this was once the mainspring of the practice. Here, as so generally in the study of human culture, the nature of a practice is not to be explained by the working of motives which move ourselves, nor is it even to be explained fully by the immediate motives of those who now put the custom into practice. It is only by historical inquiry, by finding the social concomitants and antecedents of the custom, that we can hope to understand its nature.

Further, if we inquire into the history of the practice, we must continually ask ourselves to what extent the community of practice and of idea underlying the practice depends upon a community of culture due to the movements of mankind over the earth's surface. Directly we go closely into any concrete examination of convergence, we are inevitably lead to inquiries into the history of the practice, and thus are brought into a position in which we have to consider the part played by transmission. I have looked at the matter from the point of view of the believer in independent origin, and have found that we are brought up against the idea of transmission directly we probe at all deeply. Let us now consider the matter explicitly from the standpoint of the believer in transmission, and see whither we are led.

The body of students whose work is inspired by the belief in the vast rôle played by transmission is so small, and their real activity is so recent, that there have not yet been developed those varieties of standpoint and method which will undoubtedly arise. It is, however, even now possible to see the beginning of the divergence of two paths. According to one school of advocates of transmission, the carriage of culture by a people from one place to another is a more or less mechanical process in which social customs or institutions find a new home without suffering any essential change or with such minor modifications as are necessary to adapt them to their new environment. To those who look on the transmission of culture in this way, it is difficult to see how convergence can occur. Only divergence is possible, produced by the modifications of custom or institution brought about by differences of physical or social environment.

The other path leads to a far more complicated process, in which a process of convergence is possible. To those who believe in the intimate adaptation of social institutions to the mental constitution and environment of their possessors, it is difficult, often impossible, to conceive that social institutions can ever have been transmitted in any direct manner from one place to another; and, even if this occur, it may be taken as certain that the introduction of a new form of social organization or a new religion is no simple and direct process, but one in which a new product arises as the result of introduced ideas and social practices. Every introduction is the occasion of a new growth which arises through a process of interaction between introduced ideas and practices and indigenous sentiments and institutions. If this be so, it is evident that the new institutions may sometimes diverge in different directions from the parent. But it is also possible, that in two places customs or institutions may come into existence which differ from the parent institution, but yet resemble one another through similarity either of environment or of the mental constitution of the peoples among whom the new growths take place.   In such a case we should have a similarity arising out of difference, a process to which the term convergence would be appropriately applied.   Thus, convergence is not necessarily the outcome of independent evolution ; it may be the direct result of the contact and interaction of cultures.

In illustration I will again use the practice of head-hunting and will formulate a hypothetical process of transmission according to which the custom would not have spread directly from Austronesia to America or *vice versa*, but might have been an independent growth in each place.   Let us assume the existence of a people, say in Asia, who possessed a cult of dead ancestors whom they propitiated by human sacrifices offered on such important occasions as the building of a new home or the launching of a new canoe.   So long as this people lived in their original home, the supply of old or young or infirm persons of their own community may have been amply sufficient to supply the victims.   Let us now suppose that the people are dispersed and travel widely afar in search of a new home.   The members of a migrating band will have far too high a value to be used as victims, and, if the offerings to the ancestors are to continue, the victims will have to be taken from the peoples whom they meet on the way or find already dwelling in the countries where they settle.   The capture of prisoners to be used in sacrifice will become a feature of the cultures implanted by the migrants in their new homes.

So long as victims are chosen from among themselves, there will be no difficulties about their transport to the place of sacrifice, but as soon as foreign captives are used for this purpose, it will become necessary to be content with some part of the body as the representative of the whole. If, either as an element of their own original culture, or by borrowing in the course of their journeys, the migrants came to regard the head as the representative of the body, we should have all the conditions necessary for the independent origin of the practice of head-hunting. If two parties of the people thus dispersed from their original home settled in two regions so different from one another, both in physical environment and in the character of the indigenous people, as Melanesia and America, we should have the custom of head-hunting coming into being in such diverse environments, physical and social, that the process would seem to be one of convergence. It is only by historical inquiry that we should discover the ultimate dependence of the similarity in transmission.

The conclusion to which we are thus led by an attempt to trace out the sequence of events to which convergent customs may be due shows us that the production of similarities among different peoples and in different environments may be indistinguishable on superficial examination from cases, of independent convergence, and may yet owe their general character and even their details to an origin from some common source. In ethnology, as in biology, the concept of convergence is not one with which we should ever be content as a final explanation. If we say that the occurrence of similarities of culture is due to convergence, the usage may be justified so long as we recognize clearly that we are only using the term for a social process in a superficial and inconclusive manner. The diagnosis of convergence still leaves us with the main problem unsolved. We still have to discover how far the similarity is due to the action of laws common to the mental constitution of mankind, and how far it has been produced by similarities of mental and social equipment not common to mankind at large, but the special possession of a people derived from one home who by their wanderings in different directions have come to form a common element of the widely diverse populations of places remote from one another in space and in the general nature of their culture.

My object in this chapter is to suggest that it will be useful to class together certain social processes as cases of convergence so long as we recognize clearly that we are still left with the task of discovering the mechanism to which this convergence is due. Convergence will be a useful concept in ethnology only if we recognize that the convergence may be historical or psychological, or, as will probably be found more frequently, dependent on a process which can only be fully understood when studied by the combination of the historical and psychological methods.

II

A MODERN MEGALITHIC CULTURE

(Written in 1915)

In the controversy now being carried on between the advocates of independent origin and transmission in the production of similarities of object and custom in different parts of the world, a prominent place has been taken by the rude structures of stone usually known as megaliths. These structures, and especially those known as dolmens, have so great a similarity in different parts of the earth that they furnish an excellent means by which the question of dispute may be put to the test.

More than forty years ago, Fergusson, who had then made the most comprehensive study of these monuments, was led to regard them as having had a common origin in some one part of the earth whence they had been carried by the migrations of culture, but soon after that time the belief in independent origin gradually pervaded the anthropological atmosphere and this belief became so great an article of faith that, with hardly an exception, the wonderful similarities in the megalithic monuments of different regions were regarded as products of the interaction between the human mind and its environment. This belief gained ground in spite of the vast variety of the geographical conditions of the places where megalithic monuments are found and the total absence of any evidence for specific mental similarities which could possibly have led mankind to the erection of monuments having so special a form as that of the dolmen.

During the last few years, this dogma has been thrown over by a body of students led by Elliot Smith, who has put forward a number of reasons for regarding these monuments as the work of one culture, if most of them were not the work of one migrant people.

In the opinion of an increasing number of students, the main position of Elliot Smith and his colleagues has been established, but it will be necessary to consolidate the points by much work, in which the megalithic cultures of different regions of the world are compared in detail and their points of difference explained by reference to local conditions in the places where such differences are found.

In this work two tasks are especially prominent. One is concerned with chronology. The history of the megalithic culture will not be satisfactory till we are able to place the megalithic monuments of different parts of the world, not merely in relation to one another, but in their order of time.

The second task is still more important. If the megalithic monuments of the world belong to one culture, a culture which came into being somewhere and spread thence by the migration of peoples, we can be confident that they, or rather the body of sentiments and beliefs which led to their erection, would not have travelled alone ; we can be confident that these monuments form only one element in a complex culture which was implanted in so many different regions.

The present chapter is intended as a contribution to the solution of these two problems or sets of problems. The first interest of the facts we put forward here is that they show us a megalithic culture which is still active, one in which people are now putting up rude monuments of stone, in response to the needs of their social and religious ceremonial. Moreover, there is evidence that in certain districts the megalithic culture is still undergoing modification and that the modifications are still passing from people to people, still showing that tendency to spread which must have been so strong to produce their wide diffusion over the earth. From the point of view of chronology, the interest of our communication will lie in showing that the spread of the megalithic culture is still in progress and that even the invasion of our region by the materialism and commercialism of our civilization has not yet succeeded in arresting its growth and spread. If the megalithic culture is thus still spreading it shows how cautious we should be in our attempts at chronology, while it also shows clearly that the spread of these monuments cannot be wholly the work of one people or of one age, but has been a process of gradual diffusion and infiltration which in many parts of the world has been continuously spreading a cult of peace and worship during the many centuries that western civilization has been cultivating the gospel of war and of commercialism.

The discovery of a still living megalithic culture has, however, far more fruitful and important consequences, since the study of the culture of the people who are still erecting megalithic monuments should teach us much about the history of the past.

Most of the megalithic monuments of the world were made by people who have vanished from the scene. It is only the massive and enduring character of the monuments that has permitted their survival when every other feature of the culture once associated with them has disappeared. This disappearance is not only true of our own time ; it had already taken place when man began to write the histories of his race, or had already become so shadowy as to escape the notice of those by whom these histories were written. If this culture still survives in some isolated region, even if greatly modified by conditions of time and place, it cannot but give us some clue to the long vanished beliefs and customs of the people who erected the trilithons of Stonehenge and Tonga, the pyramids of Egypt, Tahiti and America, and other megalithic forms.

What are these monuments and how far are we justified in regarding them as megalithic ?

The monuments and cultures I am about to describe are found in the northern islands of the New Hebrides. They probably exist in other parts of the archipelago, but my inquiries were limited to the northern islands and it is only with them that I deal in this chapter, and especially with the islands of Malekula and Santo and the small islands adjacent to them.

The monuments consist of structures closely resembling dolmens and menhirs, stone circles, and stone platforms. It is the structures resembling dolmens which chiefly concern us as megalithic work. These structures consist of a horizontal stone resting upon a number of vertical upright or rounded stones so as to enclose a space ; they differ greatly in form, but these differences are probably largely due to the nature of the material with which the monuments were constructed. The largest seen by me and one most nearly approaching the typical dolmen in form, stands at Nogugu on the north-western coast of Santo. In this district, the monuments are called *sua* and, in addition to the lateral stones on which the table-stone rests, have, or should have, a central stone, called *korowain-sua* or root of the *sua*, which in the only example still remaining is carved so as to resemble a phallus. In the southern part of this island, in the Isle of Tangoa and in the districts of Malo which were visited, the corresponding structures were smaller and round or square rather than long, thus departing widely from the typical dolmen. But these features are almost certainly due to the use of coral in their construction, and the circular form of the structure in many cases can safely be ascribed to the frequent use of circular growths of coral as the largest pieces of stone available. In the islands of Tangoa and in some parts of Malo, the structures have become little more than flat stones surrounded by small uprights so as to resemble a fence.

In the islands of Santo, Tango and Malo, the only stone structures which I saw were these dolmen-like monuments. In Malekula and the islands adjacent to it to the north-east coast, there was much more variety. The structures resembling dolmens were found in far larger numbers and in most cases were associated with menhirs, the menhir standing by the side of the dolmen. There were also large groups of menhirs, circles of stones surrounding sacred objects, platforms of stone and stone-images.

Except in regions where Christianity has had great influence, these structures are not relics of some past state of society, but form an integral part of the ceremonial of the people and are still made at the present time.

The social institutions with which they are especially connected are the organizations which, though not secret in the New Hebrides, have so many points of resemblance with the secret societies of other parts of the world.

The only organization of this kind of which up to the present we have had any adequate account is the *Sukwe* of the Banks Islands, accounts of which have been given by Codrington [1] and by myself. [2] The organizations of which the stone monuments of the New Hebrides form part resemble the *Sukwe* of the Banks Islands in many respects, and in many parts of Santo and Malo are known by forms of the same name : *Supwe* in Santo, and *Sumbe* and *Supur* in Malo. In other parts of Santo, the organizations are named after the cycas or *Miocle*, while in Malekula and adjacent islands, they are called *Maki*, *Mangki*, *Memgge* or *Mangge*.

These organizations form a series of grades which largely

---

[1] *The Melanesians*, Oxford, 1891.
[2] *History of Melanesian Society*, 1914, i, chap. iii.

determine the place which persons take in the social life. Each rank is attained by the performance of ceremonial which tends to become more elaborate in the higher grades of the organization, and the erection of stone structures forms a definite part of this ceremonial, being associated in most cases with the higher ranks. In the islands of Atchin and Vau whence come our most complete records, the feature by which persons are graded in rank by means of the organization has become of relatively little importance, while rites resembling those which in other islands accompany attainment of high rank have undergone great development, and form a complicated ceremonial the performance of which confers the same kind of social importance which in other islands depends upon the attainment of the higher ranks of the association.

In the *Supwe* of Nogugu in Santo, there are at least sixteen ranks, but the setting up of the dolmen-like *sua* only begins about the middle of the series at a stage called *U'u* or (*Uku* in another part of this district). Men attain new rank by killing pigs and, when doing so for the grade of *U'u*, the new member stands on newly constructed *sua*, while for earlier stages he stands upon a simple flat stone.

The attainment of the rank of *U'u* is preceded by a prolonged ceremony called *wôs*, the most definite feature of which is the drinking of kava by the old, and the throwing of boomerangs by the young men every five days. This goes on for about a year, at the end of which the new *sua* is made in readiness for the final ceremony of initiation into *U'u*.

The *sua* is also important in the ceremonial of death. Men of high rank are placed on the ground in the extended position, and the body covered by a piece of canvas. At the end of fifty days the skull is removed by the brother or sister's son of the deceased who keeps it till he takes the rank of *U'u*, when he buries the jaw-bone of his dead relative under his *sua* by the side of the phallus-like stone called the *korowaia sua.* This is done with the idea that the ghost of his relative will assist him in obtaining and killing the pigs necessary for the attainment of rank in the *Supwe.*

In Nogugu, it is possible to discern the presence of two stages in the ceremonial use of stone. The rank of *U'u* marks the change from one mode of disposal of the dead to another. The bodies of men below this rank are placed on platforms of trellis-work, while for this rank and above they are treated in the manner already described. This change in the mode of disposing of the dead corresponds with the change from the use of a flat-stone to the *sua* as the object upon which a man stands when killing his pigs for a new rank. The association of these two uses of stone with two wholly different modes of disposing of the dead suggests that the present form of the *Supwe* is due to the fusion of two elements, both practising the ceremonial use of stone.

In the southern part of Santo, stone monuments called *vota*, which corresponds to the *sua* of Nogugu, are less like a dolmen in appearance. They are used in the ceremonial of the *Supwe* in connection with the killing of pigs, but I have no knowledge of the details of the rites connected with their use. In the island of Tangoa to the south of Santo, the *vota* are said to have been used as seats by men of high rank.

III

THE PROBLEM OF AUSTRALIAN CULTURE [1]

THE question which is to form the subject of this chapter is only a special case of a problem which now occupies a foremost place in the study of human culture. Until recently, the majority of students of anthropology, and practically the whole body of British anthropologists, have based their theoretical constructions upon the assumption that the varieties of human culture now to be found in different parts of the earth are the results of a process of evolution, in which some simple group of human beings has gradually developed by contact with variety of physical environment into the highly complicated forms of such Societies as our own. It is either explicitly stated, or the conclusions of this school imply, that the lowly varieties of human culture, which are found in many parts of the world, represent either stages in the direct line of evolution from some simple beginning, or that they are offshoots of this evolution, side-tracks as it were, which have failed to reach that condition we are accustomed to regard as the highest form of human society, but have yet persisted here and there in isolated parts of the earth.

In the speculations of most of those who belong to this school of thought, it is assumed that the manners and customs of these isolated peoples furnish us with the means of studying directly the origins and early stages of human institutions.

If we examine the higher cultures of mankind, such as those

[1] Read before Section H of the British Association, 1914, Australia. Much of the material of this essay is embodied in a different form in the last essay of the book, " The Contact of Peoples."

of Europe or Asia, it is evident that they are the product of a highly complex mixture of peoples. No historian would ever think of ignoring the influence of Roman, Saxon, Dane and Norman who have all played so prominent a part in the development of the social institutions of Great Britain. But it has been hitherto assumed by many students that such mixture has been limited to peoples we know to have possessed the means and appliances for wide movements over the earth's surface, and especially upon the sea. It has seemed incredible to them that in prehistoric times there could ever have taken place such movements over the earth as those of our own age.

For long, however, there have been others whose vision of man's past history has not been thus limited. They believe that the vast movement over the earth's surface in which we and our immediate predecessors have been privileged to take part, is only the latest of a long series of similar movements, movements which have taken place far more slowly and gradually than those of which we are still the witnesses, but yet have reached as far and have had effects as great.

If such movements and mixtures of peoples have taken place, we cannot assume, when we find a social institution in a relatively simple form among a savage or barbarous people, that it represents the origin or early form of the institution in question. It may be only the degenerate survival of a highly-developed form of the institution brought from elsewhere, or it may be a special product of the interaction between a culture of a relatively high order and one of a lowly aboriginal people. Our knowledge has now progressed so far that most are prepared to accept with all its consequences the composite character of many existing peoples of the world, but there are many who still hold fast to the view that peoples are to be found who are the simple products of development from some primæval form uncomplicated by external influence.

One of the places thus chosen as an example of simplicity of culture is Australia. The work of many Australian ethnologists during the last twenty years has given us a wide knowledge of the aboriginal culture of this continent, and this knowledge has been avidly seized by the evolutionary school and made the basis of far-reaching theories of the origins of many human institutions. The relations between the Australian aborigines and animals and plants have been made the basis of more than one theory of totemism, and the origin of other human institutions and customs has been sought in the beliefs and practices of the peoples who once occupied this country. In all these theories it is explicitly stated or implicitly assumed that the Australian customs have been the outcome of the ideas and sentiments of a variety of the human race, unassisted by, and independent of, external influences. It is this concentration upon the Australian aborigines which makes the problem of the simplicity or complexity of their culture of such fundamental importance to the science of anthropology.

Now we can hardly expect to solve the problem if we attend to Australia alone. We have to compare Australian culture, not with all sorts and conditions of culture from China to Peru, as has been so much the fashion in recent times, but with examples having a definite geographical and cultural continuity with that of Australia. Here we meet our first difficulty in the apparently unique character of Australian culture, which seems at first sight to remove it from that of contiguous peoples so widely as to raise doubts concerning the validity of any such comparison. I believe, however, that Australian society is far less peculiar than is generally supposed and that the idea of its unique character has arisen, partly through concentration of attention on certain highly-specialised products of its culture, partly through ignorance of neighbouring cultures. The study of Melanesian culture, made possible by recent work, shows that there are far more elements in common between Australia and Melanesia than has been hitherto supposed. The resemblances of certain forms of Melanesian culture (especially in the New Hebrides and the Bismarck Archipelago), to that of Australian culture are in many respects so great as to leave little doubt that certain influences from without which have vitally affected Melanesia, must also have reached Australia.

The conclusions drawn from this similarity of culture are strongly supported by certain geographical considerations. The comparison of Melanesian culture with that of Polynesia and of both with the culture of Indonesia, shows that the migrating peoples which have greatly influenced the islands of the Pacific, came by way of the Malay Archipelago. This is a view about which there is no disagreement. The migrant peoples from the West who have thus influenced Melanesia and Polynesia travelled on the sea. Bodies of hardy and skilful navigators have succeeded in taking, not only themselves, but also many of their possessions, their domestic animals and their food-plants, to remote islands of the Pacific. It is probable that the main route of this migration lay north of New Guinea, but even if this were so, it is most unlikely that there should have been none to try a more southern route, and that a mass of land so vast as Australia should have been untouched by peoples who reached Easter Island, New Zealand and Madagascar. Further, if we concede the exclusively northern direction of the migration, we know beyond all doubt that the migrants turned the south-eastern corner of New Guinea and passed westwards, certainly as far as the Fly River. It is again most unlikely that this westward movement of the migrants should have stopped at the flat mangrove swamps of the Fly River, and should not have been deflected southwards by the islands of Torres Strait to reach the shores of Australia.

L

The situation of Australia is such that only by a miracle can it have escaped the influences from the West which reached the neighbouring islands. If the migrant peoples who have taken so great a part in the formation of the culture of Melanesia also settled in Australia, the nautical character of the migration enables us to draw certain conclusions concerning the nature of their settlement. Nor were seafarers so enterprising likely to have been content to invade Australia at one point only, but would have coasted far in search of suitable settling-places. One reason why so many students have been blind to the presence of external influence in Australia is that they have pictured the process as the sweeping of an invading host across the continent. The history of Australian culture becomes far easier to understand if there has been a gradual infiltration of small bodies of seafaring peoples at many points on the coast, not merely on the more accessible western and northern shores, but all along the eastern and even the southern coasts. There is much in the culture of Australia which it becomes possible to link with that of neighbouring regions, if small bodies of migrants settled at many points and passed on their culture to the interior, partly by their own journeys, but still more widely by the movements of the native peoples whom they influenced.

This view is in conflict with the widely received opinion that Australia has been altogether peopled from the north by means of ancient land connections with New Guinea, an opinion which has received its chief support from the frail and apparently primitive nature of the canoes of Australia. We know, however, that in Oceania the canoe has wholly disappeared, and in islands where one would have thought the canoe essential to the existence of the people. It is, therefore, no great difficulty that canoes sufficiently seaworthy to bring migrating peoples from Indonesia should have degenerated on a continent, where the canoe is not an essential element of culture, into the fragile vessels which the Australians now possess. Defective means of navigation cannot be raised as an argument against the presence of seafaring peoples, whose influence in neighbouring regions has been so great.

The complexity of the culture of any area can only be fully established when it has become possible to formulate a scheme of its history in harmony with those of neighbouring areas of allied culture. Any historical scheme which attempts to account for the nature of Australian culture must be in harmony with the schemes of the history of Melanesia and New Guinea, and must also be brought into line with the more remote areas of Polynesia and Indonesia. Any association of culture-elements which is ascribed to a given people in Melanesia should also be found in Australia, and where there are differences, it ought to be possible to show that these are due to differences in the physical or social environments of the two places. The object of this paper is to state a problem rather than attempt a solution to it. It will be possible, however, to take one element of culture and show how far a cursory study of its features illustrates the nature of the general problem.

There are few features of culture in which the conservatism of mankind shows itself more strongly than in rites associated with the disposal of the dead. It is the intimate relation of the rites of death with the most sacred beliefs and sentiments of mankind, which accounts at once for the extraordinary persistence of features of these rites and for the success with which immigrant peoples succeed in carrying their rites into a new home. Wherever we find diversity of funeral rites, we may safely conclude that there has been diversity of culture.

A people who move from one home to another of widely different physical character, may be driven to practise new forms of death-cults, and this may happen without contact with any other people.   Apart from this, we can be confident that changes in the rites of death arise only through the most definite social needs, and it is the duty of any who believe in the spontaneous origin of new rites of death to show what those social needs have been.

The nature of the funeral rites of the Australian aboriginal should thus furnish us with a guide to the solution of the problem we are now considering.   If Australian culture be simple, we should expect to find only one mode of disposal of the dead, or at the most such variants of one method as can be explained by such differences of physical environment as would act as stimuli to change.   As a matter of fact, there are few areas of the world which present so great a variety of funeral rites.   Nearly all the chief modes of disposal of the dead are present.   There is interment in the extended and contracted positions (both with and without a coffin, the coffin being a canoe or part of a canoe, or a log of wood to represent a canoe).   There is also the practice of preservation above the ground on a platform or in a tree, and there are cave-burials and cremation.   Further, there are complex forms in which some two of these modes of disposal are combined.   These different rites are not limited to definite regions, but may occur in districts close to one another, and in such a distribution as seems wholly inexplicable by differences of surroundings, but just such as might be expected if the different methods had been introduced, not at one spot to spread thence over the continent, but by peoples who have landed at many different points.

Moreover, this local diversity seems to be especially pronounced near the coasts just as might be expected if the different methods have been brought by peoples who have travelled on the sea.   This great diversity of funeral rites, and the mode of distribution of the various forms are only sufficient to provide a general case for complexity. To establish that case, it will be necessary to show that these various modes belong to different aboriginal and immigrant peoples, and if, as I have supposed, the immigrants into Australia are the same as those who have reached Melanesia, any scheme formulated to explain the Australian facts must be in general agreement with the Melanesian scheme, and should place its component elements in the same order of time. In widely separated parts of the world it may sometimes happen, through the blending of cultures, that an element of culture which is the earlier in one place may be the later in another, but in regions so near to one another as Australia and Melanesia, we cannot be content unless the time-order of its immigrant cultures be the same. By reliance on criteria of different kinds, on the mode of distribution, on associations with other elements of culture and the use of different methods by chiefs and commoners, I have found it possible to construct a scheme for Melanesia, in which the order of the immigrant cultures has been from interment in the contracted and sitting position, through cave-burial, preservation and interment in the extended position, to cremation as the latest product of external influence. If this scheme of Melanesian culture is to hold good, it will be necessary to show that the time-order in Australia corresponds with it. At present we have two schemes of the complexity of Australian culture before us, those of Dr Graebner and Father Schmidt. These two schemes agree 'in many respects with one another, but differ very widely from that to be expected if there is any truth in my scheme of Melanesian history.

The complexity of Australian culture which is suggested by the ritual of death is not one which has been produced by the local influence of Malay or Papuan, but has been due to several successive settlements whose influence has spread widely over the Continent ; and these influences have not been slight or superficial, but account for much which is generally held to be distinctive of Australian culture, for its different forms of mutilation, for its beliefs in the reincarnation of the dead, for its totemism and to a large extent for its matrimonial classes, and the dual form of its society.

IV

THE DISTRIBUTION OF MEGALITHIC
CIVILIZATION

(This brief chapter is the contribution made by Dr Rivers to the discussion on *The Influence of Ancient Egyptian Civilization on the World's Culture* at the meeting of the British Association in Manchester in 1915.)

I THINK I can best contribute to this discussion by describing how the new evidence and new arrangement of old evidence brought forward by Prof. Elliot Smith and Mr Perry have influenced my own attitude towards the problems connected with the history of megalithic monuments.

Ever since I became interested in the contact and blending of peoples as the dominant factor in human progress, I have expected that the megalithic monuments of the world would provide us with the first convincing demonstration of the importance of these factors. I have now for several years been convinced that the ideas underlying the construction of megalithic monuments had their origin in some one part of the world, whence they spread to other parts, but until the publication of recent evidence I hesitated to follow Elliot Smith in his conclusion that the home of the megalithic culture was Egypt. His paper on the evolution of the dolmen was sufficient to establish the very close relations between the dolmen and the Egyptian mastaba : but it did not seem to me sufficient to prove conclusively that the mastaba was the prototype and original ancestor of the world-wide dolmen.

It may be instructive to dwell for a moment on the reasons which led me to hesitate. One was undoubtedly a prejudice against Egypt as the birthplace of custom and belief, owing to the many wild and uncritical attempts which have long been made to derive practices of remote parts of the world from Egypt, attempts which we now see to have often been in the right direction, though the truth was obscured by the method in which its demonstration was attempted.

A far more potent cause of my hesitation, however, was the great simplicity of the process assumed by Elliot Smith. I have so keen a sense of the complexity of human progress that I distrust a simple explanation. If we find a feature of culture common to two regions, there are always two possible lines of interpretation in addition to that by independent origin. The feature in question may have travelled from one place to the other, or it may have reached both localities from some third place where it had come into being. When, therefore, it became obvious through the work of Elliot Smith that the mastaba and dolmen were genetically related to one another, my first inclination was to regard the mastaba as the result of a special line of development in ideas which elsewhere produced the dolmen, and I preferred to remain in suspense concerning the original home of these ideas rather than accept their origin in Egypt.

Such remained my state of mind till the Meeting of the Association in Sydney in 1914, when Professor Elliot Smith demonstrated the close resemblance in the details of Egyptian and Papuan mummification, a demonstration which has been made still more complete in a publication of the Literary and Philosophical Society of Manchester, issued in 1915. This work [1] shows that the practices used by the people of Torres Strait in order to preserve their dead, agree with those of Egypt in no less than seven points of detail. If we accept the independent origin of mummification in Torres Strait, we are forced to believe that, in a climate most unsuited for

---

[1] Published in book form as " The Migrations of Early Culture," 1915.

such experiments, the rude savages of these islands invented a procedure which took the highly civilized Egyptian many centuries of patient research to attain. I prefer not to adopt such a miracle as a scientific explanation, but to accept completely the view that there had been a direct transference of culture from one place to the other, and in this case there can, of course, be no shadow of doubt that the movement was from Egypt to Torres Strait and not in the reverse direction. I no longer hesitate to believe that the group of customs and beliefs forming the complex most suitably known as megalithic, developed in Egypt and spread thence to the many parts of the world where we find evidence of its existence at the present time.

The opening address has dealt with two chief questions. Who were the people who carried the Egyptian practices over the world? What was the composite of the group of practices so carried? I propose to deal only very briefly with the latter question.

The correspondence of the details of Papuan mummification with those of Egypt at the time of the XXIst dynasty has led Elliot Smith to fix upon the 8th century B.C. as the date of the wandering which carried this complex over the earth, and I am prepared fully to accept the view that an extensive migration occurred at that time. I hesitate, however, to accept the whole list of practices and beliefs which he has given us as belonging to that special wave of migration. This list rests mainly on the fact of common distribution, and there is one feature of the mode of distribution of the megalithic complex which introduces a possible source of error into the problem. There can be no doubt that the complex of customs which included the construction of megaliths was carried by sea, the distribution being especially definite on islands and along coast-lines. Such a distribution may well have been due to more than one migration.

As I have pointed out elsewhere,[1] the evidence from Melanesia suggests that more than one stream of megalithic influence reached that remote region, and as we get to know more of other parts of the world, I expect we shall find similar evidence in favour of the double or even multiple character of the megalithic culture. The facts seem to receive a natural explanation if the maritime movements which carried the megalithic culture from Egypt and its neighbourhood were of long duration. We gather that the movements became discontinuous as they spread outwards from the centre of distribution, so that distant regions such as Melanesia and America were reached in successive waves, separated perhaps by considerable intervals of time. If this were so, it is evident in the first place that we have no right to conclude that the migration which left the confines of Europe, Asia, Africa about the 8th century B.C. was the first of these world-wanderings, and certainly must we keep in mind the influence of later movements. The recent work of Mr Layard and myself in the New Hebrides has shown that movements of the megalithic culture have taken place quite recently, probably during the last century. The long delayed progression in these remote islands is probably only an extreme example of a process which characterizes the transmission of culture into regions widely remote from the centre of distribution. It would take too long to attempt, from this point of view, any analysis of the long list of customs assigned by Professor Elliot Smith to the megalithic culture. I must be content to suggest these considerations which point to the necessity of such analysis.

So far I have dealt only with the contribution of Professor Elliot Smith to this discussion[2]. Great and far-reaching as its consequences are, it has a worthy companion in the paper

[1] *The History of Melanesian Society*, 2 vols., 1914.
[2] *Discussion on the Influence of Ancient Egyptian Civilization on the World's Culture*, Report of the Br: Assoc; Manchester, 1915, p. 667.

of Mr Perry[1]. Here again I hope that I may be allowed to consider the matter in relation to its influence on my own line of thought. Ever since I realized the great importance of migration in the history of human progress, the subject has been obscured by our almost total ignorance concerning the motives which led mankind to undertake such ambitious journeys. I may remark that these ancient travellers reached parts of the world which have only come within the ken of our own geographers during the last two or three centuries. To take only one instance, the Torres Strait, which we now know to have been reached by Egyptian influence, were wholly unknown to our civilization till they were traversed less than three centuries ago by the Spaniard whose name they bear.

Until recently the view which seemed to afford the best explanation of the waves of culture which have spread over the world is that there has been a series of disturbances in some parts of the world which drove the inhabitants to seek new homes on a large scale. The waves of culture which seem to have reached even so distant and isolated a region as Melanesia suggested a series of such distributions, perhaps at some such intervals as are suggested by Professor Petrie's stimulating book, *The Revolutions of Civilization*. Further, the work of Huntington [2] suggested that the place from which these migrations started was Central Asia, and the cause the periodical drying up of that continent. It still seems possible that this process may account for some of the waves of culture which have travelled over the earth's surface, but Mr Perry's evidence seems to me to dispose of the theory that the motive force was purely geographical. The force was attractive rather than propulsive, viz., the love of wealth, which is still the most potent factor in immigration. The maps of distribution shown by Mr Perry reveal with a clearness

---

[1] *Ibid.*, p. 669.
[2] *The Pulse of Asia.*

which has few, if any, parallels in the history of ethnology, that the carriers of the Egyptian culture three thousand years ago were impelled by the same motives as those which lead the people of our own time.

Mr Perry's demonstration not only provides the cause of the wandering which is the special subject of our discussion, but, what is perhaps even more important, it shows in a most striking way the continuity of thought and action upon which alone a true science of ethnology can find a sure foundation.

V

LAND TENURE IN MELANESIA

In his account of Melanesian land tenure, Dr Codrington notes [1] the general agreement in the whole character of landed property throughout Melanesia, and especially how precisely alike in different places is the nature of property in land reclaimed from the bush. The special features of land tenure in which this close agreement appears are that, where land has been cultivated for a long period of time, its ownership is vested in a matrilineal group, and that when a piece of land is regarded as the property of an individual man it passes at his death to his sisters' children, whereas land which a man has himself cleared is inherited by his own offspring. Codrington mentions several cases where land is held in common, but does not dwell strongly on the feature of common ownership, his attention being especially directed to the problems of descent and inheritance which have occupied so prominent a place in the attention of students of early society.

Codrington discusses the question of communal marriage fully, [2] but appears to have paid much less attention to facts bearing on communism in property. In the island of Mota, which is one of the places whence Codrington drew much of his information, I worked [3] out the mode of transmission from generation to generation of a plot of land from the time that it was originally reclaimed from the bush, and obtained a striking example of the strength of the communal sentiment.

[1] *The Melanesians*, Oxford, 1891, p. 61.
[2] *Ibid.*, p. 27.
[3] *The History of Melanesian Society*, Cambridge, 1914, vol. i, p. 55.

I was told that those parts of the plot which had been assigned by the original clearer to his children as their individual property were the subject of continual dispute, while that part of the original estate which had remained the common property of the descendants was never the cause of any difference of opinion.

An important feature of Codrington's account is that his information was derived chiefly from three islands, Mota, in the Banks group, Florida, in the Solomons, and Pentecost, in the New Hebrides, in all of which the social organization is on a matrilineal basis. This makes it possible that the close agreement which Codrington found in the nature of land tenure in these widely separated parts of Melanesia may be associated with the matrilineal character of the three societies.

Melanesia is commonly regarded as the seat of characteristic mother-right, but I have shown [1] that even where descent in the social group is strictly matrilineal, the mode of transmission in other respects is often in the male line. Thus, throughout Melanesia, so far as our available knowledge goes, some kinds of property pass from a father to his children, while other kinds are inherited by the sisters' children, and wherever there is definite succession to rank in Melanesia, this takes place in the male line. Melanesia has an extraordinary variety of states intermediate between mother-right and father-right. Moreover, in parts of Melanesia, father-right exists in a pure form. Children belong to their father's social group, inherit his property and succeed to his rank if he has any. It so happens that the two islands in which I have been able to study land tenure most closely are examples of this state of father-right, and my first aim is to show how close a resemblance there is in the character of landed property between these places and those parts of Melanesia where mother-right flourishes.

[1] *Op. cit., The History of Melanesian Society*, vol. ii, p. 90.

The two patrilineal islands whose land tenure I am about to describe are Ambrim in the New Hebrides and Eddystone Island in the western part of the Solomons. In order to understand the nature of the ownership of land in these places, it will be necessary to give a brief general account of their social organisation. I will begin with Ambrim, where my account [1] comes especially from the Sulol district at the western end of the island, south of the great volcano.

In Ambrim, the unit of society is the village with its surrounding district. The people of the village and district form a definite social group which is exogamous, a man of one village having to take his wife from another. Within the village there are a number of groups called *vantinbül*, each of which consists of a group of near relatives in the male line, together with the children of the sisters of its members, but not the children of these children. Thus, membership of a *vantinbül* passes in the male line continuously, but descendants in the female line remain members of the *vantinbül* for one generation, when the membership lapses. Probably it would be more correct to say that the sisters' children have certain rights in connection with the *vantinbül* of the mother, rather than that they are actually its members, rights which may be illustrated by the rules concerning land to be now described.

The situation concerning uncultivated land in Ambrim is of precisely the same kind as that recorded by Codrington in the matrilineal parts of Melanesia. So long as land is uncleared and uncultivated, no one takes any interest in it ; the people are only interested in the trees on the land. If a person wishes to clear and cultivate a portion, he can choose any part without question, but the ownership of any trees on the portion he cultivates would not be affected ; the trees would remain the property of their original owners. In order to

---

[1] This account was obtained during a visit to the New Hebrides in 1914, the full record of which has not yet been published.

cultivate the land he would have to cut down trees, but he would not disturb those of economic value, such as coconuts, or the bearers of other edible produce, and these trees would remain the property of their original owners. When a European wishes to buy uncleared land, he has to discover who owns the trees on the land ; and when he has bought these trees he will have satisfied all the claims of the people to the land.

Each village has its own cultivated land, generally spoken of as " the land of the village." Though thus regarded in one sense as the property of the whole village, different portions are held to belong to different *vantinbül*. The land of the *vantinbül* can be used by any of its members, who can take fruit or other produce from any part of it and cut down trees growing on it. Thus, all the children of a man can use their father's garden, and the daughters continue to do so after their marriage and transmit this right to their children, but at the death of these children ownership or usufruct lapses. Though the people are now patrilineal we seem to have here an indication of coexistent inheritance by the sisters' children. The study of Ambrim ceremonial points clearly to a former state of mother-right,[1] and this right of persons to use their mother's land is probably a relic of the earlier line of inheritance.

A point emphasized by the people when talking about the ownership of land is that if a man has cultivated a piece of land exclusively by his own labours, its produce can nevertheless be taken by any other members of his *vantinbül* without asking permission and without letting the cultivator know that they have done so. The produce may also be taken freely by other members of the village not of the cultivator's *vantinbül*, but only after asking permission. It was stated, however, that such permission would never be refused. In

---

[1] See *Journ. Roy. Anth. Inst.*, 1915, vol. xlv, p. 229.

practice, therefore, the produce of the land is free to the whole village, but there is the definite distinction that members of the *vantinbül* take without asking leave, while the other members of the village must go through the formality of asking permission of a member of the smaller group in whom ownership is theoretically vested.

It is clear that in practice there is communism in the ownership of land and in the use of land, only limited by the obligation in certain cases to ask leave, rather, it would appear, as a matter of good manners than of imperative right.

From our point of view it would seem that such communism would make it possible for a man to live without working, and that the island would provide a paradise for the slacker. I inquired carefully into what would be done in such a case. It was clear that if a man was lazy and never did a stroke of work in cultivating the gardens, he would be allowed to take produce freely from the land of his *vantinbül* without asking leave of anyone. But I could not find that such a case ever occurred owing to the social disapprobation which such conduct would entail.

If all the members of a *vantinbül* were to die, the land, already regarded in one sense as the property of the village, would become so in the sense that no individual or group in the village would have any special rights to its use. It would remain common for a time, probably until it had become overgrown, and then people would gradually begin to plant trees on it, and after a time would claim the ground on which the trees were growing for their *vantinbül*, and thus the land would again become the property of one or more of these groups.

If all the members of a *vantinbül* in the male line died out, but women of the *vantinbül* still had living children, these would use the land till their death, but their children would have no further rights and could not hinder its becoming the property of their mother's village.

One other point of interest may be noted. In the language of Ambrim when people speak of different objects, they indicate the nature of the ownership, whether individual or communal, by the use of different possessive pronouns, single, dual or plural. In the case of land the plural possessive is always used, a man speaking of his garden as *samemchul tel*, our garden. Sometimes a man might make a very small garden exclusively by his own labour and might then call it *sak tel*, my garden ; even then, however, he could not keep its produce for his own use, but it could be taken by any other members of his *vantinbül*.

The social structure of the island of Eddystone in the Solomons, where I obtained my other facts about land tenure,[1] though definitely patrilineal, differs in many respects from that of Ambrim. In giving an outline of its social organization it is first necessary to note that though Eddystone is only a small island not more than two miles long and only a quarter of a mile broad in the middle, it has four districts inhabited by groups of people who are largely independent of one another, and were certainly formerly still more independent. Within each of these four districts the most important social group in relation to land tenure is the *taviti*, which consists of persons related through both father and mother, the limits of the group being determined genealogically. A man regards as his *taviti* all those with whom he can trace genealogical relationship other than by marriage. The group thus corresponds with that which among ourselves is composed of relatives by blood as opposed to relatives by marriage, but the limits of the Melanesian group are more definitely defined, and the group has more definite social functions.

[1] This account forms part of the work of the Percy Sladen Trust Expedition of 1908.

Within the group of *taviti* two distinctions are made : a man distinguishes between his *taviti* of his own district and those belonging to other districts ; and he also distinguishes between *taviti* related to him through his father and *taviti* through his mother.   These two distinctions often cover one another, for the usual way in which a man comes to have *taviti* of a district other than his own is by the marriage of his father with a woman of another district.   At the present time marriages are mostly between men and women of the same district, and formerly this was even more habitual.   If all the marriages of a man's ancestors had taken place within his district all his *taviti* would be of his own district, unless for any reason a man had gone to live in a district other than his own.

I pass now to the description of land tenure, and the first point to note is that in ordinary conversation a man speaks of a piece of land or garden as " my land " or " my garden," and a superficial observer might easily suppose that the island afforded an example of the individual ownership of land.   On going into the matter more deeply, however, I found that a man distinguished between land which he called his through his father and land which had come to him from his mother, and that in the first case he shared his rights to the and with the *taviti* of his father and in the second with the *taviti* of his mother.   When a man said that a piece of land was his, and had come to him from his father, it was found that any of his *taviti* through his father could make a garden on this land, and that *taviti* through his mother could similarly make gardens on the land he had inherited from his mother.   Moreover, in each case the *taviti* could take produce from land he had cultivated, and it was especially emphasized that both the making of gardens and the taking of produce did not require the leave of anyone, but was an unquestioned right.

If, on the other hand, *taviti* belonging to a district different from that in which the land was situated wished to make a garden or take produce, they would have to ask leave of one of the group of owners, but here, as in Ambrim, it seemed that permission was never refused. As already stated, there is reason to believe that formerly marriages only took place within the district and that men of one district did not take wives from another, in which case all *taviti* would have belonged to the same district and no *taviti* would have had to ask for leave.

This account shows that, though the social group in which the ownership of land is vested differs in character between Ambrim and Eddystone, there is a striking similarity between the two places in the nature of the common ownership, and even in such a detail as the distinction between the use of land or produce with and without permission. As I have already said, both these places are patrilineal, Eddystone, however, differing from Ambrim in that it was not possible to discover any evidence pointing to an earlier state of mother-right.

I propose now briefly to examine Codrington's evidence from other parts of Melanesia where mother-right still flourishes, to see how far their systems of land tenure agree with those of Ambrim and Eddystone so far as their communistic character is concerned. In the island of Florida in the Solomons, property is never held absolutely by the individual, but is vested in the *kema*, the matrilineal totemic clan. In the Banks Islands, Codrington states that gardens are individual in that an owner can be found for each piece. He distinguishes between ancient hereditary ground and land recently reclaimed from the bush. In the former case, Codrington states that a group of relatives do not hold the property in common. My own work in Mota showed [1] that this is not strictly accurate, and that part of a piece of land

[1] *Op. cit.*, i, p. 56.

cleared in recent times may remain common to all the descendants of the clearer. I have already mentioned the striking fact that while quarrels about the portions individually owned are frequent, disputes never arise about the portion owned in common.

In Pentecost in the New Hebrides, Codrington [1] only refers to the mode of inheritance by the sister's son and does not mention common ownership, but I was told [2] that the ownership of all kinds of property was formerly vested in a group called *verana*, a subdivision of the moiety [3] which forms the primary social group of the greater part of that island.

I have already pointed out that Codrington was especially interested in the mode of inheritance, and that his references to common ownership are scanty and vague ; but such facts as he gives, supplemented by my own inquiries, point to a state of affairs very similar to that found in Ambrim and Eddystone Island.

I have not so far mentioned Fiji, an archipelago which, though largely Melanesian, has undergone, probably as the result of Polynesian influence, so special a development that it is customary to put it in a category apart. Nevertheless, here again, as we learn from Lorimer Fison, [4] the ownership of land is communal. Ownership is vested in joint tribal owners called *taukei*, the social group concerned being the *matanggali*, which corresponds closely with the local group of Melanesia. We find also an interesting distinction which I have not met in other parts of Melanesia. A member of any *matanggali* may cut grass or reeds from a plot of arable land which is not actually in use, but he may not turn the soil on any plot other than his own. It seems that the people distinguish between the use of products of the soil and the use of the soil itself.

[1] *Op. cit.*, p. 67. [2] *Op. cit.*, i, p. 209.
[3] Many communities in Melanesia and elsewhere possess what is termed the Dual Organization ; they are divided into two divisions termed moieties, the members of which usually intermarry.
[4] *Journ. Anthrop. Inst.*, vol. x (1881), p. 332.

I have now to describe an aspect of land tenure in Melanesia which I have not so far mentioned, viz. the place of chiefs in relation to the land. Fison has pointed out that the whole problem of the nature of Fijian land tenure is greatly complicated by the claims of the chiefs to ownership of the land. There is no question that the institution of chieftainship in Fiji has been greatly modified in recent times as the result, partly direct, partly indirect, of European influence, and its importance in the life of the community has been greatly enhanced. As a result of their increased importance, the Fijian chiefs have claimed rights in the land inconsistent with the common ownership which Fison believed to be the ancient custom of the country. The state of other parts of Melanesia, where chieftainship has been modified to a smaller extent, clearly supports Fison's contention. In some of the places from which examples of land tenure have been given, such as the New Hebrides and the Banks Islands, the institution of chieftainship cannot properly be said to exist, the place of chiefs being taken by the old men or by men of high rank in certain special organizations.[1] In the Solomons, however, where hereditary chieftainship is a definite institution, it is clear that the chiefs have no special rights of any kind in connection with the land. More than this, Codrington records [2] a striking case of landless chiefs at Saa in the island of Mala or Malaita. The hereditary chiefs of this place are descended from immigrants who came in about eleven generations ago. Though the descendants of the indigenous inhabitants are now few in number and of the lower orders, they are still the owners of the land, and the chiefs are content to have land allotted to them which they can use for their gardens.

The different islands of Melanesia from which the foregoing

---

[1] See *History of Melanesian Society*, ii, p. 99.
[2] *Op. cit.*, p. 50.

examples of land tenure have been taken differ greatly in their general culture, including their social organization. The Banks Islands and the New Hebrides are the seat of a characteristic form of the dual organization of society which still exists in some parts of the Solomons [1] and with little doubt formerly existed in Florida,[2] but no trace of its presence is to be found in Eddystone. Totemism, though of a somewhat aberrant form, occurs in Florida, but is completely absent on Ambrim and Eddystone, while the Banks Islands and Pentecost only present features which may be distantly connected with this form of social organization. The Banks Islands and Ambrim are the seats of highly complex and more or less esoteric organizations, and a similar organization formerly existed in Florida, but no trace of their presence can be detected in Eddystone. It is a striking fact that this remarkable diversity should be accompanied by so great an agreement as characterises the ownership of land and the rules concerning its use. This close agreement suggests that the communistic attitude towards landed property goes back to an early stratum of the population and to an early phase in the history of Melanesia. This view is strongly supported by the relation of chiefs to the land. There is no question but that the case of landless chiefs which Codrington records from Malaita is only a recent example of a process which has been general in Melanesia, the chiefs in general being the descendants of immigrants.[3] It is, therefore, of great significance that chiefs should have no special privileges in relation to land or should even, as at Saa, be wholly destitute of a share in its ownership.

I have confined my attention to the ownership of land, but an examination of other forms of property would bring out many features of common ownership, though less definitely

---

[1] See C. E. Fox, *Journ. Roy. Anthrop. Inst.*, 1919, vol. xlix, p. 120.
[2] *History of Melanesian Society*, ii, p. 72.
[3] *Op. cit.*, ii, p. 325.

than in the case of land. The wide agreement in the nature of Melanesian land tenure affords strong support to the view put forward in *The History of Melanesian Society* [1] that an early (not necessarily the earliest) phase in this history was one in which all forms of property were held in common by a social group, and that in spite of influences which have produced the great diversity of Melanesian custom and institution, this communistic aspect has remained distinctly present in relation to land.

It will have been noticed that on more than one occasion I have mentioned the ownership of trees as an institution independent of the ownership of the land on which the trees are growing. This Melanesian custom has excited much interest but it has been little studied, and I propose now to consider it with the aim of discovering whether it may help us to understand Melanesian land tenure and its history. I will begin by recounting the facts, beginning with those recorded by Codrington in the matrilineal parts of Melanesia.

He states that in the Banks Islands property in trees is distinct from that in land and goes to the planter's children, while, as we have already seen, land often passes to the sisters' children. When in Mota I found, however, that if a man planted a tree on the land of one to whom he is unrelated, he can only transmit his right in the tree to his son if money is paid to the owner of the land, and I give an instance of a dispute about the ownership of a nut-tree which had arisen out of a special departure from the usual law of inheritance. [2] I found also that when there is no relationship between the planter of a tree and the owner of the land, the permission of the latter must be obtained and that as a rule he only permits one tree to be planted by a person in this way.

Similar customs prevail in Florida. [3] If a man plants a

[1] Vol. ii, p. 384.
[2] *History of Melanesian Society*, i, p. 52.
[3] Codrington, *op. cit.*, p. 62.

useful tree on the land of a friend, it goes to the planter's son, but that the right is not absolute is suggested by the statement that it will so pass only if the landowner remains friendly. Similarly, a man can plant trees on his own land expressly for the use of his sons, so that at his death they pass to them, while the land itself passes to his sisters' children.

In the patrilineal island of Ambrim I found a somewhat different state of affairs. As elsewhere, the people seemed to be especially interested in the ownership of trees, an interest strikingly exemplified in the sale of uncultivated land, where the buyer satisfies all claims to the land when he buys the trees standing on it. Similarly it was said that when land had become common to the village through the extinction of a *vantinbül*, the process by which the land again became the property of a *vantinbül* began with the planting of trees upon the land. I did not hear, however, that it was definitely the custom to plant trees upon the land of a *vantinbül* other than that of the planter. If I am right that this custom does not exist, its absence is probably to be connected, partly with the extent to which the common ownership of trees is still recognized, partly with the fact that the Ambrimese have a special mode of acquiring individual ownership of trees by means of rites forming parts of the ceremonial organizations called *Mangge* and *Temärkon*. The *Mangge* is an organization in which a man gradually rises in rank through a process of initiation accompanied by ceremonial which grows in complexity with every rise in rank.[1] One of the features of each initiation is that certain trees are set aside for the individual use of the new member of the grade, the trees thus devoted to individual ownership being indicated by means of a branch of the cycas or wild cane. Trees may also be appropriated to individual use by means of taboo marks. Both in this case and when the taboo forms part of the ritual of the *Mangge*,

---

[1] See article " New Hebrides " in Hastings' *Encyclopædia*.

it is believed that infringement causes sickness due to the anger of the ancestral ghosts.

In the ceremony called *Temärkon*, which takes its name from the bull-roarer, the case is somewhat different. Those initiated into the use of this instrument smear certain trees with black pigment taken from their bodies and set up crotons by these trees, which indicate that their produce may only be used by those who have been initiated into *Temärkon*.

In Eddystone Island a man can not only plant a tree upon the land of another person or another group of *taviti*, but it is not necessary to ask the permission of the owner or owners of the land. The trees are the property of the planter, and at his death pass to his children. There was at one period of my work a doubt whether people ever objected to having trees planted in this way on their land, and it was said that sometimes they would cut them down. This might lead to a fight. The only concrete case of which I could learn, however, was of a special kind. In this case, a fight in which many were wounded took place between two villages because certain trees had been cut down. The man who had destroyed the trees in this case, however, was not the owner of the land on which the trees were growing, but the destruction was the work of a number of young men who were having what we should call a " rag " in the course of a ceremony. I could not hear of any case in which the owner of a piece of land had ever so far objected to trees being planted by others on his land as to cut them down.

Eddystone Island differs from many parts of Melanesia in that it possesses a definite currency, used not only in ceremonial, but as part of the general economic life, and sometimes a man would buy from another the trees on a piece of land, the land remaining the property of the vendor. Useful trees and especially the coconut, areca-nut and betel-vine, could also be tabooed for the special benefit of an individual by means of certain rites, called collectively *Kenjo*, in which the trees were protected by a taboo mark imposed with verbal and manual rites of various kinds. There were many varieties of these taboos, each belonging to a small group of persons who alone knew the rites or in whose hands they were alone efficacious. As in Ambrim, one who took fruit thus protected would suffer from disease or other misfortune, each variety of taboo bringing a special kind of disease as penalty for its infringement, which, again, as in Ambrim, was ascribed to the action of ancestral ghosts.

In Fiji also, fruit-trees are often held by persons who do not own the land. Here there is the special feature that though the owner of the tree uses its fruit, he may not cut it down without the permission of the owner of the land.[1] In one case, it was said that the owner might cut down the tree provided his axe did not touch the soil, but he would not be allowed to dig up the tree by its roots. This case suggests that the ownership of trees is free of any implication of ownership of the soil in which the tree is growing.

The general account of Melanesian land tenure has suggested that the communistic nature of the ownership of land goes back to an early stage in Melanesian history; and the special laws connected with the ownership of trees seem to be just such as might come into being as the result of compromises between an indigenous people who owned the soil and settlers from without. If the indigenous people had a deep-lying sentiment concerning the ownership of land and would not part with any of it, even to immigrants who became their chiefs, the needs of the settlers would seem to have been met, in part at any rate, by allowing the strangers to own trees.

The development of a custom of this kind would be

[1] L. Fison, quoted by Codrington, *op. cit.*, p. 61.

especially easy to understand if the immigrants had brought with them seeds or slips of fruit-trees unknown to the indigenous inhabitants. I have little evidence concerning the nature of the trees owned independently of the land, except that the practice seems to be especially frequent in the case of the coconut.

In those cases, however, in which trees or their fruit are appropriated to individuals by means of religious ceremonial, I have definite evidence of the prevalence, or even limitation, of the custom to trees of certain kinds. Thus, in Eddystone Island the only trees protected by the special taboo called *kenjo* are the coconut, areca-nut and betel-vine. Similarly, in Ambrim the cycas, a plant of great importance in ceremonial, is especially used to taboo the coconut. There is every reason to believe that betel-chewing is a practice of relatively late introduction into Melanesia, and it is probable that the areca-nut and betel-vine utilized in this practice were introduced at the same time. It is also probable that the coconut has similarly been introduced from without.

One piece of evidence from Ambrim lends strong support to the view that the appropriation of trees or their produce to individual use by means of religious ceremonial is the result of external influence. In Ambrim, there is a definite tradition that the *Mangge* and *Temārkon*, the two organizations with which the practice is associated, have been introduced in relatively recent times into the island, while other ceremonial organizations are much older, if not indigenous.[1] It seems as if the introducers of these organizations utilized their religious rites as a means of obtaining special privileges inconsistent with the communistic sentiments of the people to whom the organizations had been brought. It would seem that both this case as well as the individual ownership of trees generally

---

[1] *Journ. Roy. Anthrop. Instit.*, 1915, vol. xlv, p. 230.

are to be regarded as compromises,[1] arising out of a conflict between the communistic sentiments of an indigenous people and the desire of settlers from without for the individual ownership to which they were accustomed in the place from which they had come.

[1] *Folk-lore*, 1921, vol. xxxii, p. 25.

VI

THE DISAPPEARANCE OF USEFUL ARTS [1]

THE civilized person, imbued with utilitarian ideas, finds it difficult to understand the disappearance of useful arts. To him it seems almost incredible that arts which not merely add to the comfort and happiness of a people but such as seem almost essential to his very existence should be lost. He assumes that the loss is only to be accounted for by such factors as the total lack of raw material or the occurrence of some catastrophe which has wiped out of existence every person capable of practising the art. The object of this tribute to Professor Westermarck is to show that arts of the highest utility have disappeared in Oceania and to suggest that the causes of the disappearance are not simple, but that social and magico-religious, as well as material and utilitarian, factors must be taken into account. I shall deal with three objects : the canoe, pottery, and the bow and arrow.

The Canoe

It might be thought that, if there was one art of life which would have been retained by people living in small groups of islands, it would be the art of navigation. Even putting aside the need for intercourse between the inhabitants of different islands of a group and with the inhabitants of other groups, one would have thought that its usefulness in obtain-

[1] Reprinted with the permission of Prof. Westermarck, from *Festskrift Tillagnad Edward Westermarck*.

ing food would have been sufficient to make people strain
every resource to the utmost to preserve so necessary an
object as the canoe. Nevertheless we have clear evidence
that in two places in Oceania the canoe has once been present
and has disappeared.

In the Torres Islands (not to be confused with the islands
of Torres Strait), the people have at present no canoes and
in order to pass over the narrow channels, which separate the
islands of their group from one another, they use rude cata-
marans of bamboo. These craft are so unseaworthy that
they are of little use for fishing ; how little is shown by the
fact that in order to catch the much prized *un* (the *palolo* of
Polynesia) the people stand on the reefs and catch the worms
with a net at the end of a long pole.

It is quite certain that we have not to do in this case with
people who have never possessed the canoe. The Torres
Islands form only an outlying group of the Banks Islands
which in their turn form a continuous chain with the New
Hebrides, and the general culture of the Torres islanders is
so closely allied to that of neighbouring peoples, and there is
such definite tradition of intercourse with them, that, even if
there were no more direct evidence, we could be confident
that the people must once have shared the prevailing outrigger canoe of this region with their neighbours. Direct
evidence, however, is not wanting. Dr Codrington records [1]
that the canoe-makers had died out and that the people had
in consequence resigned themselves to doing without an art
which must once have taken an important place in their daily
avocations.

While the canoe has thus disappeared in the Torres group,
there is evidence that it has degenerated in the adjacent Banks
Islands. The canoe of these islands is now a far less seaworthy and useful craft than it must once have been. There

[1] *The Melanesians*, 1891, p. 293.

are clear traditions of former communications with the Torres and New Hebrides, if not with more distant islands, but now the canoes only suffice for journeys within the Banks group and are not even good enough to fulfil this purpose completely. The canoe of Mota cannot be trusted to take its people to the island of Merlav which forms the southern limit of the group. Further, Dr Codrington records [1] that at Lakon, a district of Santa Maria, one of the largest of the Banks Islands, the people for a time went without their canoes, though, unlike the Torres islanders, they had re-learnt the art.

It is clear that this disappearance or degeneration of the canoe is not due to modern European influence. The canoe had already disappeared in the Torres Islands when Dr Codrington was in Melanesia, and this was not long enough after the settlement of Europeans to allow the loss to be ascribed to this cause.

The other place in Oceania where we have evidence of the disappearance of the canoe is Mangareva (Gambier Islands). When this island was first visited by Beechey,[2] he found the people using large rafts capable of carrying twenty men, together with smaller craft of the same kind; and yet, as Friederici has pointed out,[3] there is one fact which shows that these islanders had formerly possessed the canoe. The Mangareva people call their raft *kiatu*, a widely distributed word in the Pacific for the outrigger of the canoe. We can be confident that this word indicates a direct relation between the Mangareva raft and the ordinary Polynesian canoe. Even if it would be rash to conclude that the raft is the direct descendant of the outrigger of an ancient canoe, we can be confident that the natives of Mangareva were once acquainted with the canoe, but had it no longer when their island first

---

[1] *Loc. cit.*

[2] *Narrative of a Voyage to the Pacific*, 1831, i, 142.

[3] *Beiträge z. Völker- und Sprachenkunde von Deutsch-Neuguinea*, Berlin, 1912, p. 247.

became known early in the last century. When Beechey visited Mangareva, the people sailed their rafts and could do so much with them that it would not be correct to say that they had lost the art of navigation, as may be said about the Torres Islanders. Nevertheless the art must have been very inferior to that which was given to them by the possession of the canoe.

Pottery

Pottery is less essential to the life of an islander than a canoe. Yet its convenience must be so great that its manufacture would seem to be an art most unlikely to disappear.

The distribution of pottery is one of the most remarkable features of the material culture of Oceania. In southern Melanesia, it is now found only in two places, New Caledonia and Espiritu Santo (usually called Santo), and then, passing northwards, we do not meet with it again till we come to the Shortland Islands, Bougainville and Buka, and then it disappears again to reappear in New Guinea. Eastwards, it is found in Fiji, but is totally absent from Polynesia.

Its distribution, however, was once more extensive. Fragments of pottery are found scattered about in Malikolo [1] and Pentecost,[2] in neither of which islands is pottery now used, and in Malikolo the people have a myth to explain the presence of the fragments. Further, pottery has been found buried at considerable depths in two places, and promises through its indestructibility to become in these distant islands as important a guide to past history as in the older world. In Lepers' Island (Omba), Glaumont has found [3] coarse potsherds lying nine feet below the surface, and in Ambrym,[4]

[1] Somerville, *Journ. Anth. Inst.*, 1894, vol. xxiii, p. 378.
[2] Joly, *Bull. d. l. Soc. d'Anth.*, Paris, 1904, Sér. V., t. V., p. 366.
[3] *Voyage d'Exploration aux Nouvelles-Hébrides*, Niort, 1899 (abstract *Globus*, 1899, vol. lxxvi, p. 228).
[4] Joly, *op. cit.*, p. 365.

pottery has been found accompanying an ancient burial. We have here clear evidence of the use of pottery over an extensive region in only one corner of which it is still made.

Similar discoveries of ancient pottery have been made in New Guinea.[1] Here, pots are still made in the districts where this ancient pottery has been found, but in south-eastern New Guinea, the ancient pottery is far superior to that now made, though similar to it in several respects. The modern pottery which most nearly approaches the old in character is that used in Murua (Woodlark Island), as a receptacle for the bones of the dead. If, as is probable, this modern pottery is the direct descendant of the old, we may note that it has survived in its completest form, not for a utilitarian purpose, but as part of the ritual of death.

There is thus clear evidence that pottery has disappeared from some islands where it was once in regular use, and that in others where pottery is still used, the art has fallen far below its former level of excellence.

The Bow and Arrow

There is definite evidence that the bow and arrow was once a far more widespread and important weapon in Oceania than it is at present.[2]

In Polynesia, it is only definitely known to have been used as a weapon in Tonga [3] and Samoa.[4] In Tahiti, the use of the bow in war is doubtful,[5] but it was used to shoot at a mark in sport and it is difficult to understand the existence of archery as a sport if the bow had not once had a more serious

[1] Seligmann and Joyce, *Anthropological Essays presented to E. B. Tylor*, 1907, p. 333, and Pöch, *Mitt. Anth. Gesellsch*, Vienna, 1907, vol. xxxvii, p. 67.
[2] This evidence has been recently fully set out and discussed by Friederici, *op. cit.*, pp. 119-133.
[3] Mariner's *Tonga*, vol. i, p. 283 and vol. ii, p. 287.
[4] Wilkes, *Narrative U.S. Exploring Expedition*, 1845, vol. ii, p. 151.
[5] See Appendix A, p. 208.

use. In other parts of Polynesia, the bow is used in sport especially to kill rats, and also to shoot birds and fish for food. Here again, there can be little doubt that these uses are only survivals of a time when it was employed as a weapon. What little doubt remains is dissipated when we find that the word for the bow of Polynesia is often *pana*, *fana*, or *ana*, forms of a widespread word for the bow in Oceania and used in places where the bow is the chief weapon.

In Melanesia the conditions are much as in Polynesia, the bow and arrow being used as a toy or to shoot birds and fish in places where there is evidence of its former use in war.

In New Britain the bow is only used in war by the Kilenge people of the north coast,[1] and, since they obtain it from the people of New Guinea, it might be thought that it has only recently been introduced. The bow is used in war in the middle of New Ireland but the people at the southern end use it only to shoot pigeons.[2] In New Hanover,[3] the bow and arrow is said to be now unknown and in the Admiralty Islands it has hitherto only been known as a toy, though the Hamburg Expedition has recently discovered a bow once used in war.[4]

There is clear evidence, however, that in some of these islands the use of the bow in war was once more general. The ancient voyagers record that the natives of these islands shot at them with arrows and there is some evidence in favour of a progressive diminution in the importance of this weapon.[5] Again, though the bow was till recently used in war in the British Solomons,[6] it was certainly a less important

---

[1] Danks, *Rep. Austral. Assoc.*, 1892, p. 619; Kleintitschen, *Die Küstenbewohner der Gazelle-Halbinsel*, Hiltrup (preface dated 1906), p. 212; Brown, *Melanesians and Polynesians*, p. 324; and Friederici, *op. cit.*, p. 119.

[2] Stephan and Graebner, *Neu-Mecklenburg*, Berlin, 1907, p. 51.

[3] Strauch, *Zeitsch. f. Ethnol.*, 1877, vol. ix, p. 54.

[4] *Globus*, 1909, vol. xcv, p. 103.

[5] See Appendix B, p. 209.

[6] Codrington, *Melanesians*, p. 304.

weapon than when the islands were visited by the Spaniards two centuries earlier.[1]

In many parts of New Guinea, and especially among the people who speak languages of the Melanesian family, the bow and arrow is now absent, or used only as a toy or to shoot birds. In this case there is more justification for the view that the bow has been introduced recently, for in parts of German New Guinea, the bows and arrows used by the coastal people to shoot birds are obtained from the natives of the interior,[2] while on the south coast of British New Guinea they are obtained from the people of the Papuan Gulf.[3]

In German New Guinea, however, a fact has been recorded which points clearly to the bow and arrow being a survival rather than a recently introduced element of culture. Pöch [4] found that the Monumbo living on the coast opposite Vulcan Island in German New Guinea do not use the bow and arrow. They have, however, a word for the bow in their language, and in their marriage ceremony the bride holds in her hand a symbolic bow and arrow, this ceremonial use pointing unmistakably to the ancient importance of the weapon thus symbolized.

In British New Guinea, again, the storing of the bow and arrow in the *marea* or clubhouse among the Roro [5] suggests that this weapon is an ancient possession of the people, and this is supported by the fact that even the Papuan tribes from whom the bow is obtained apply to it terms which are almost certainly Melanesian. In New Guinea, as in Melanesia, there is thus reason to believe that the bow and arrow was once a more important element of the culture than it is at present.

---

[1] *Discovery of Solomon Islands* (Hakluyt Soc.), 1901, vol. i, p. lxxvii and pp. 24, 34, 47, 50, 57, etc.
[2] Friederici, *op. cit.*, p. 120.   See p. 112.
[3] Seligmann, *Melanesians of British New Guinea*, pp. 93, 215.
[4] *Globus*, 1903, vol. xciii, p. 141.
[5] Seligmann, *op. cit.*, p. 229.

Having now established the fact that in certain parts of Oceania there have been lost three arts the utility of which would seem to make their disappearance most unlikely, I proceed to consider to what causes this disappearance is to be ascribed. I will consider these causes under three heads, material, social and magico-religious.

Material Causes

The most obvious cause of the disappearance of an art, however useful it may be, is the absence of the raw material out of which it is made, and I have first to consider whether the disuse of the canoe and of the bow in many parts of Oceania may have been due to lack of suitable wood and that of pottery to the want of clay.

There are certain features of the art of canoe-making in the Pacific which suggest the lack of raw material as a possible cause. There are islands of the Pacific where there are no trees from which a dug-out canoe could be made and, the people have to depend on the arrival of driftwood. Further, this dependence on driftwood may be necessary even in islands where there are suitable trees, owing to the implements of the people being incapable either of cutting down a tree of sufficient size or of hollowing it after it has been felled. It is not difficult to see how a people may allow their implements to degenerate till they are incapable of felling or hollowing trees so that after a time they become dependent upon driftwood, and that then some change of current or other cause may allow so long a time to elapse without arrival of suitable wood as to explain the loss of the art.

There is no reason, however, for supposing that this has been the cause of the disappearance of the canoe either in the Torres Islands or Mangareva. The Torres Islands are well wooded and their implements are not notably, if at all, inferior to those of neighbouring groups of islands where the canoe is still made. Again, the picture of the Mangareva raft in Beechey's book shows that the natives were able to use large planks of wood, and absence of suitable material may here also be put on one side.

There is no reason whatever for supposing that absence of suitable material has played any part in the disappearance of the bow, but with pottery the case is different. The geological character of many of the islands of the Pacific shows that they must be quite devoid of any material from which pots could be made, and the absence of raw material is probably a most important, if not the essential, factor accounting for the absence of pottery from Polynesian culture. Absence of clay, however, will not explain the disappearance of pottery in Melanesia and the ancient pottery of Lepers' Island was covered by many feet of clay-like earth which would probably have been suitable for the manufacture of pots if the art had not disappeared through some other cause. Though absence of raw material may have caused the loss of the potter's art in Polynesia, it cannot explain its disappearance in Melanesia, nor can it explain the loss of the canoe and of the bow and arrow.

Material and utilitarian motives of other kinds have been suggested to account for the disuse of the bow and arrow as a weapon. Gill [1] has suggested that the eastern Polynesians did not use the bow in war because their arrows could not pierce the folds of cloth with which they covered their bodies. Even if this were a sufficient motive in eastern Polynesia, it would not explain the disuse of the bow elsewhere in Oceania. Again, Peschel [2] has suggested the absence of land-mammals as the cause of the disuse of the bow and arrow in Polynesia, pointing out that the bow is a weapon which requires con-

---

[1] *Life in the Southern Islands*, London (preface 1876), p. 28.
[2] *Völkerkunde* 6th edition, Leipzig, 1885, p. 187.

stant practice in peace in order to ensure accuracy of aim in war. The use of the bow and arrow in sport throughout Polynesia seems, however, to provide the necessary element of practice and the archery of Tahiti must almost certainly have had such practice as its original motive.

Peschel explained the disuse of the bow and arrow in New Britain and New Ireland in the same way, ignoring the fact that there is no such difference in the nature of the fauna of different parts of the Bismarck Archipelago and New Guinea as will account for the use of the bow in some places and not in others. Further, Peschel seems to have forgotten the fact that the bow is the prevailing weapon of southern Melanesia where land-mammals are even more scarce than in those parts of Melanesia from which the bow is absent.

A more probable motive for the disuse of the bow in Polynesia has been suggested by Friederici,[1] who points out its unsuitability to the physical conditions of Polynesian warfare. He believes, almost certainly with right, that the bow was a prominent, if not the chief, weapon of the ancestors of the Polynesians. The warfare of the Polynesians is conducted in canoes or on shores affording little cover from the wind and Friederici has himself seen how the strong winds of the Pacific make the arrow a fluttering and harmless missile. He suggests that the bow was the weapon of a people accustomed to fight in the bush who found it ill adapted to the more open character of the islands of Polynesia.

This factor, however, will not explain the disuse of the bow as a weapon over large regions of Melanesia where bush-warfare exists. Nevertheless, it is possible that the disappearance of the bow has been due here also to the special nature of the warfare. The leading principle of the strategy

[1] *Loc. cit.* ; also *Mitt. d. Verein f. Erdkunde*, Leipzig, 1910 (1911) p. 165.

of many parts of Melanesia is the use of surprise. The object of an invading party is to come to close quarters and destroy the enemy in the early morning, while he is still asleep. The importance of this mode of warfare cannot, however, fully account for the disappearance of the bow and arrow, for this weapon is still used by some of the people who practise this war by stealth. It is probable that the causes of the disappearance of the bow and arrow in so many parts of Melanesia have not been purely material, but that other motives have been in action.

Social Causes

A second group of factors which may bring about the loss of useful arts are social. Many of the objects used in the everyday life of Oceania are not made by any member of the community, but their manufacture is confined to special groups of craftsmen. Thus, in Tonga and Tikopia, canoes are only made by certain men called *tufunga* who are succeeded in this occupation by their sons. Though in Tikopia a man can become a *tufunga* through his own efforts, the obstacles in the way of his success are very great and the craftsmen thus form a body limited in number, definitely distinguished from the rest of the community. It is only necessary for such a limited body of men to disappear either as the result of disease or war or through some natural catastrophe, to account for the disappearance of an art. As we have seen, there is evidence that this dying out of skilled craftsmen has been the cause of the disappearance of the canoe in the Torres Islands, and Seligmann and Strong [1] have recorded the dying out of skilled craftsmen as the cause of the disappearance of the art of making stone adzes in the Suloga district of Murua (Woodlark Island). The dying out

[1] *Geographical Journal*, 1906, vol. xxvii, p. 347.

of skilled craftsmen within a community is thus established as a cause of the loss of useful arts.

This factor, however, will only explain a localized loss here and there. It will explain the loss of the canoe on isolated groups of islands, but it will not account for the absence of the bow and arrow or of pottery over large areas of Oceania. The skilled craftsmen would not be likely to die out simultaneously among all the peoples of an extensive area.

In certain parts of Oceania there are, however, conditions which make the extensive loss of useful arts more intelligible. Useful objects are often made only in certain places whence they spread over a large area by means of trade. Thus, the people of the Papuan Gulf obtain their pots from the Motu and Koita round about Port Moresby, and trade in pottery is also found among the Massim.[1] Again, in New Caledonia pots are said to be made only in three places.[2] The extermination of the people who made pottery by warfare or by some natural catastrophe might thus be limited to a small region and yet it might lead to the disappearance of the use of pottery over large and even remote regions. There is some reason to suppose that a catastrophe of a volcanic character may have led to the loss of pottery in the northern New Hebrides. The fragments of pottery found in Lepers' Island lay under two layers of soil, the deeper of which consisted of scoriæ. In this region where volcanoes are even now active,[3] it is possible that the use of pottery throughout an extensive region was discontinued by the destruction of some special people from whom the pottery was obtained. It is even possible that the pottery of Santo may have been introduced later into a region from which pottery had been

[1] See Seligmann, *op. cit.*, pp. 96 and 526.
[2] De Vaux, *Rev. d'Ethnog.*, 1883, vol. ii, p. 340.
[3] Volcanoes are still active in Ambrim and Lopevi and volcanic activity has not yet exhausted itself in Lepers' Island. Codrington, *Melanesians*, p. 14.

eliminated many ages before by a volcanic catastrophe. We should have in such a case a combination of material and social factors. If pottery were once made in every island and district of the northern New Hebrides, it is very unlikely that any volcanic catastrophe would have wiped it out completely ; but the limitation of the art to one district is a social factor which makes intelligible such an effect of the material agency. The material factor, acting alone, would not have abolished the art, but in combination with the limitation of the manufacture to special tribes, it would enable a localized catastrophe to destroy an art over a wide region. Even this combination of causes, however, would not destroy an art over such extensive regions of Oceania as some of those in which useful arts have disappeared.

It is possible that social causes may have assisted the utilitarian motives suggested by Friederici as the cause of the disuse of the bow and arrow as a weapon. In many parts of Polynesia, if not generally, fighting had largely a ceremonial character, the killing of a man on either side or even the drawing of blood being sufficient to put an end to a fight. In such a condition, strictly utilitarian motives would count for very little and thus a process by which one weapon was changed for a less deadly one would be facilitated.

Again, among a people so advanced as the Polynesians, it is a question whether the mere play of fashion may not have had a great influence. If war were the deadly process it is with us, it is most unlikely that a weapon capable of killing at a distance should give way to one which can only be used at close quarters, but if war is largely ceremonial, it is possible that the bow and arrow may have been supplanted by the club. The great development of the club in Polynesia, its manifold development in form and ornament, show how great a part it has played in the interests and affections of the people. It does not seem unlikely that the club may have so become the fashion at one stage of Polynesian history and so excited the æsthetic, and perhaps the religious, emotions and sentiments of the people, that the bow and arrow ceased not merely to be an object of interest ; it ceased to be used at all for the serious business of warfare and persisted only for the relatively unimportant purposes of shooting birds, rats and fish or for the pure sport of archery.

Useful arts may also disappear through the influence of an immigrant people. The contact of two peoples has social consequences of a complicated character in which elements of the material culture may be involved. It is unlikely that immigrant influence would ever lead people to discard such useful objects as pottery and the canoe, but it is probable that it has played a part in the disuse of the bow and arrow in Melanesia. It is even possible that the change of fashion I have supposed to have occurred in Polynesia may have been connected with the presence of a new ethnic element in the population.

Religious and Magical Factors

In the last section I have suggested that religious factors may have assisted the development of the club in Polynesia and thus helped to bring about the disappearance of the bow and arrow as a weapon. There is another religious factor which may have worked in the same direction. People whose highest hope it is to die in battle, to whom this end opens the way to a future life in a special paradise, are not likely to be swayed by utilitarian motives in their choice of weapons. If the bow and arrow had a great superiority as a weapon, and if war were waged in earnest, we could have trusted to natural selection to ensure its survival, but in the absence of such superiority, the Polynesian contempt for death may have had a share in its disappearance.

It is also possible that religious or magical motives may have assisted the loss of useful arts dependent upon the dying out of special craftsmen. To our utilitarian minds there may seem to be a serious objection to the view that useful arts have disappeared through the dying out of craftsmen. We can readily understand how such a factor would produce a great falling off in workmanship and ornamentation, but from our point of view it would seem most unlikely that people would stand idly by and allow the disappearance of arts so useful as those of making pottery and canoes. Nevertheless, we have found that arts have disappeared for this reason and it remains to discover why. In many parts of Oceania, an art practised by a special group of craftsmen is not a mere technical performance but has a definitely religious character and may be regarded as a long series of religious rites. It is not enough to be able to make a canoe, but you must also know the appropriate rites which will make it safe to use it for profane purposes without danger from ghostly or other supernatural agencies. To go in a canoe which has not been the subject of such rites would be to put oneself into the midst of all kinds of hidden and mysterious dangers. In Polynesia, this religious character of crafts is shown even in the terms applied to those who practise them. The *tufunga* of Tonga and Tikopia is only one form of the *tohunga* of the Maori, the *tuhuna* of Tahiti, the *taunga* of Mangaia, the *tahunga* of the Low Archipelago and the *kahuna* of the Hawaiian Islands. Most of these words are used both for priests and craftsmen,[1] thus pointing clearly to the religious character of the occupations they follow. In combination with rites which so often accompany the process of manufacture, this common nomenclature suggests that the disappearance of useful arts through the dying of craftsmen may not have been due solely, or even chiefly, to the loss of their manual skill

---

[1] Cf. Christian, *Eastern Pacific Lands*, 1910, p. 162.

but that the quenching of their spiritual power, the *mana* of Oceania, may have been another and most potent factor.

I have no case in which I can definitely show that a useful art has disappeared from religious or magical motives. I wish rather to direct attention to the possibility of such motives in order that workers in the field and theorists at home may not be content with obvious utilitarian explanations of the loss of useful arts. I can, however, cite a case where a ceremonial custom has disappeared which shows how such motives as I have assumed are able to abolish important elements of culture. A variety of circumcision, more suitably termed incision, is a widespread Polynesian custom, but it is absent in certain islands such as Penrhyn, Niue, Pukupuku and Manihiki. Gill [1] believes that the custom was once practised in these islands, but has disappeared owing to the absence of the red quartz which is invariably used in neighbouring parts of Polynesia to perform the operation. If Gill is right, we have here a case in which a people have allowed an important rite to lapse rather than carry it out in a manner other than that hallowed by custom. If many of the arts of Oceania are at the same time religious rites, we have in the disappearance of incision a suggestive example of the kind of mechanism whereby useful arts may also have disappeared.

It is in the case of the canoe that we have the most definite evidence of the religious character of the manufacture of a useful object. In the case of pottery, I know of no such evidence, though our knowledge of this branch of Oceanic technology is very meagre. Melanesian arrows, however, have certain features which suggest a magico-religious character which may well have played a part in their disappearance. Not only is the Melanesian arrow often tipped with human bone, but it may have a human or animal form

---

[1] *Rep. Austral. Assoc.*, 1890, vol. ii, p. 327.

which would suggest a magico-religious character even if we did not know of rites designed to give efficacy to its flight. Though the material and social factors I have considered may be sufficient to account for the disuse of this weapon over large areas of Oceania, we should even here not shut our eyes to the possibility that some part in the process may have been played by magical or religious factors.

I can now consider briefly some problems of general interest towards the solution of which the conclusions of this paper may contribute.

My own interest in the subject has come directly out of my attempt to carry out an ethnological analysis of Oceanic culture. If movements of people have carried cultures over wide regions of the globe, it is inevitable that some of the elements of these cultures must disappear and thus there will be lost links in the chain of evidence. In any attempt to analyse a cultural complex, it will be often necessary to assume such disappearance ; and the probability and stability of any analytic scheme will be greatly promoted if one is able to assign motives for the disappearance, either from physical features of the environment, or from social or magico-religious features of the culture.

I hope that I have made it clear that in studying the history of culture we must be prepared for changes not to be accounted for by the likes and dislikes of the civilized and almost incredible from the utilitarian point of view. We must be very cautious in assuming that elements of culture are so useful or so important that they would never be allowed to disappear. If islanders can lose the canoe, what features of culture can we safely say can never be lost ?

A second most important aspect of my subject is one in which the loss of the canoe is especially concerned. In many regions of Oceania and in other parts of the world, islands are now to be found inhabited by people whose present means of transportation are wholly insufficient to have brought them from the nearest land.   In dealing with such problems, it has sometimes been assumed that under no circumstances is it credible that people could ever lose the art of navigation, and it has therefore been concluded that the islands must have been peopled when they were connected with some continent by a connecting bridge of land.   On similar grounds it has even been supposed that scattered islands are the mountain-peaks of submerged continents, of whose people the natives of the islands are the survivors.   Thus Giglioli,[1] starting from the assumption that the frail canoes of the Tasmanians could never have brought them from Australia, has argued that the Tasmanians must have reached their island when it was connected with the mainland.   Accepting Giglioli's statement [2] that no case is known in which people have lost the art of navigation, Howitt [3] has adopted the supposed passage of the ancestors of the Tasmanians by dry land.   Again, the culture of Easter Island has led some to suppose that it is one of the mountain-peaks of a pacific continent.   The grounds for such hypotheses and conjectures are swept away if it be established that even an art so useful as that of navigation can disappear.

Another way in which use has been made of the supposed impossibility of the loss of the art of navigation is in ascribing an indigenous character to the culture of certain regions. Thus, Mr Joyce [4] has lately argued against any influence of people from the Pacific Ocean upon South America on the grounds that along the whole of the coast of South America nothing but the most primitive raft was found.   The facts I have brought forward deprive this argument of its cogency, though it may be noted that the absence of the canoe is only

[1] *I Tasmaniani*, Milano, 1874.
[2] *Op. cit.*, p. 133.
[3] *Native Tribes of South-East Australia*, p. 9.
[4] *South American Archæology*, 1912, p. 190.

one of several features which Mr Joyce believes to point to the indigenous nature of the Andean culture.

Lastly, I cannot forbear from pointing out an allied aspect of human culture which points in the same direction as the special subject of this article.   Quite as striking as the loss of useful arts is the extraordinary persistence of elements of culture which seem to us wholly useless, and perhaps are so even to those who seem so careful to preserve them.   This persistence of the useless combines with the disappearance of the useful to make us beware of judging human culture by purely utilitarian standards.   I have perhaps in this paper gone beyond the limit warranted by my evidence in assigning the loss of useful arts to religious motives.   I have done so without misgiving, however, because I am sure that I cannot be far wrong in bringing forward views, hypothetical though they be, which will put us on our guard in estimating the motives which guide the conduct of peoples with cultures widely different from our own.   I hope that the facts brought forward in this paper have been sufficient to show that utilitarian motives are less important in determining the course of the ruder stages of man's history than we suppose them to be among ourselves.

APPENDIX A

The Bow in Tahiti

The only early visitor who records the use of the bow and arrow as a weapon is Bougainville [1] who gives the bow, the sling and a kind of pike as the weapons of the Tahitians. Cook only mentions the sling, pike and club, while Wallis expressly states that though the Tahitians use the bow and arrow, the arrow is only fit to knock down a bird, not being

---

[1] *Voyage round the World,* 1772, p. 253.

pointed, but only headed with a round stone.[1] Wilson [2] records that the bow and arrow were never used in war but only in sport ; the people shot " against each other, not at a mark, but for the greatest distance." The statements of Wallis and Wilson are confirmed by later authorities. Ellis [3] says that bows and arrows are never used except for amusement, and Gill [4] states that throughout eastern Polynesia bows and arrows were used for sport, not for war.

The Bow in New Britain and New Ireland

Since the value of the evidence for the use of the bow and arrow as a weapon in New Britain and New Ireland has been disputed, it may be useful to cite it here. In the earlier half of the eighteenth century, Behrens [5] records that the natives of New Britain shot at Roggeveen's expedition with arrows, as well as with lances and slings. Later in this century, Bougainville records [6] that the natives of New Britain attacked his ship with stones and arrows. Again, in the earlier part of the last century, Lesson [7] does not record the bow and arrow among the weapons of New Ireland, but in another place,[8] when speaking of the bows and arrows of Buka, he says that they were like those of New Ireland and New Britain. From Lesson's account, it seems that in the earlier part of the last century the bow and arrow was still used as a weapon, though it took so small a place beside the lance, club

---

[1] Hawkesworth, *Account of Voyages*, London, 1773, vol. i, p. 244 and vol. ii, p. 488.
[2] *A Missionary Voyage to the Southern Pacific Ocean*, London, 1799, p. 368.
[3] *Polynesian Researches*, vol. i, p. 299.
[4] *Life in the Southern Islands*, London, 1876, p. 28.
[5] *Reise durch die Süd-lander und um die Welt*, Frankfurt u. Leipzig, 1737, p. 151.
[6] *Voyage autour du Monde*, 2nd ed., Paris, 1772, T. ii, p. 225.
[7] See Duperrey, *Voyage autour du Monde*, 1826, T. i, p. 528.
[8] *Op. cit.*, T. i, p. 98. See also Atlas, Plate 24.

and sling, that he did not enumerate it among the weapons of the people.

The definite statements of the travellers of the eighteenth century, however, can leave no doubt about the more ancient use of the bow and arrow as a weapon and the evidence of Behrens is peculiarly valuable in that he mentions both " Pfeilen " and " Wurf-Pfeilen," showing that he did not confuse arrows with lances either in observation or memory.

The evidence suggests that the bow and arrow was becoming a less important weapon during the interval between the visits of Roggeveen and Duperrey, and that this process has continued and led to the total disuse of the bow and arrow in war.

Stephan and Graebner [1] discount the value of the evidence of Behrens and Lesson and suppose that Lesson confused New Ireland with Buka, although the way in which the essential fact is recorded makes this most improbable. More recently, Graebner [2] has cited the statements of Behrens and Lesson as examples of untrustworthy evidence and as instances of a mistake liable to be made when dealing with widely-distributed objects. The example has not been well chosen ; it would be difficult to find an ethnographical fact with better credentials. If the statements of three independent eye-witnesses [3] are not to be trusted, where are we to turn for satisfactory evidence ?

---

[1] *Neu-Mecklenburg*, pp. 7 and 51.
[2] *Methode der Ethnologie*, Heidelberg, 1911, p. 48.
[3] Graebner appears to have overlooked the evidence of one of the three, Bougainville.

VII

THE DOUBLE CANOE [1]

EVERY one who has travelled between Australia and Europe by the canal route will remember the interesting experience of the first sight of the catamaran of Ceylon. Ceylon furnishes an outlying example of a vessel which is specialized in Oceania and occurs also on the continent of Australia. It has two forms. In one form, of which the Singhalese canoe is an example, there is an outrigger only on one side of the boat, the single one ; while in the other, the double outrigger, one on each side. Each outrigger consists of two chief parts, a log of wood that rests on the water, which I shall call the float, and a structure by means of which the float is attached to the body of the canoe. The body of the boat itself is usually a dug-out, the sides of which may or may not be raised by the addition of planks. Adopting the nomenclature proposed by Dr Haddon, I shall call this attachment the outrigger boom or simply the boom.

The problem that I have to consider is the evolution of these forms of vessel, and I shall first confine my attention to the single outrigger. In the area of distribution of the outrigger canoe, does there exist any other form of vessel allied to the single outrigger canoe ? Such an ally is to be found in the double canoe, in which two canoes are fastened together side by side, forming a vessel similar to the one which came into transient use some years ago in the hope that its stability would add to the comfort of passengers across the English

[1] Read at the 1914 Meeting of the British Association in Australia.

Channel. The first problem before us is to consider whether there is any relation between the single outrigger canoe and the double canoe. A connection between them becomes highly probable when we find that the outrigger float often has the form of a canoe, making the outrigger canoe in fact a double canoe, in which one of the pair is much smaller than the other. Further, the definite genetic relation between the two constituent elements of the double canoe becomes almost certain when we find that the constituent elements of the double canoe are rarely, if ever, of the same size, and that the smaller of the pair receives the same name as the float of the outrigger. Very frequently the body of the outrigger canoe and the larger canoe of the double vessel are called by some form of the word *vaka* or *waga*, while the smaller member of the twin canoe and the float of the outrigger canoe are known by some form of the word *sama*.

Three possibilities suggest themselves. First, it is possible that the float of the outrigger suggested the second canoe, and the fancy of the people led them to fashion the float so as to make the resemblance greater. Secondly, the outrigger canoe may have been derived from the double-canoe by the gradual degeneration of one element of the double vessel. Thirdly, the double canoe may have been evolved from the outrigger canoe, the float first suggesting a second canoe, as in the first possibility I have suggested, and this fancy produced a vessel whose size, stability and strength led to its general adoption as a means of locomotion, especially for long journeys. The first of these possibilities should, I think, be kept in mind, but I do not think it worth serious discussion, and I shall deal here only with the other two alternatives.

The idea that the outrigger canoe is derived from the double canoe has been put forward by Stephan and Graebner in their book on Neu-Mecklenberg. It has the *a priori* advantage that it explains the origin of an object which it is

difficult to imagine as a simple invention by deriving it from
the device of lashing two canoes together, the idea of which
we might expect to have occurred to man even in a relatively
low stage of culture.[1]   The alternative view that the evolution
has been in the opposite direction has recently been put forward by Friederici.[2]   It has the disadvantage that it still
leaves us with the unsolved problem of the origin of the
outrigger. One of the chief arguments put forward by
Friederici in favour of his views is that if the double canoe
had been the original form, we should have expected the two
canoes to be of the same size, but, as a matter of fact, one is
always smaller than the other, this pointing to the derivation
of the smaller from the float of an outrigger. Friederici has
here ignored an important factor in the manufacture of the
Oceanic canoe.   The idea that people would naturally make
their double canoes symmetrical implies that they have a
large choice of trees for their purpose.   We know, however,
that in many parts of the Pacific the only available material
is obtained from the tree-trunks brought by the chance of
wind and current, and in these cases it must only be very
exceptionally that trees of equal size will be available.   Even
if the trees are cut down from the forest, it would only occur
exceptionally that the trees chosen for this purpose would be
found, when felled, to have their available parts of the same
length.   Friederici's argument being thus inconclusive, to
say the least, let us inquire whether there is any other evidence
on which to base a conclusion.

I will take first the distribution of the two forms of vessel.
The single outrigger is found widely in Polynesia and Melanesia
with an extension to Australia : it becomes less frequent as

[1] (At the time Dr Rivers made this assumption he was not aware
of the fact, to which Professor James H. Breasted called attention three
years later (*Journal of Egyptian Archæology*, vol. iv, 1917, p. 174) that
double floats were in use on the Nile more than fifty centuries ago.
G. E. S.)

[2] *Op. cit.* See p. 196.

one passes westward through the Malay Archipelago, probably owing to its having been supplanted by the double outrigger, and then once more it becomes the usual type of vessel in Ceylon and the Maldive Islands.

The double canoe, on the other hand, is now only found in Polynesia and Fiji. It is generally accepted that the ancestors of the Polynesians came from the Malay Archipelago, and since the outrigger exists in this archipelago, it follows from the hypothesis of the derivation of the outrigger from the double canoe that this form of canoe must once have existed in the archipelago. The limitation of the double canoe to a culture that is known to have been derived from that of the Malay Archipelago, and its absence in this region itself would be perfectly natural if the double canoe has been a special development of the outrigger canoe in Polynesia, probably in response to a need for ocean-going vessels in distinction from the coasting-vessels, which would be sufficient for a migration that hugged the coast-lines of the thickly-distributed islands of the Malay Archipelago. Not only is the distinction of the double canoe thus consistent with the origin of the double canoe from the outrigger, but we are able to point to a need which would have acted as a stimulus to the discovery of the new form. We must not shut our eyes, however, to the possibility that the double canoe may once have been present in the Malay Archipelago or some other place in the path of migration of the ancestors of the Polynesians, and that it has disappeared elsewhere owing to the later introduction of other kinds of vessel, including the double outrigger. Though the limitation of the double canoe to Polynesia suggests its relative lateness, and therefore its derivation from the double outrigger, the facts are capable of a different explanation. It is therefore necessary to look still further afield for evidence.

I propose now to consider whether we are helped in our

quest by the study of nomenclature.   Until lately, language
has been chiefly used by the ethnologist as if it were a product
of human nature which stood in little or no relation to man's
other activities, and thus was to be studied for its own sake
with little reference to other elements of culture.   We are
only now beginning to realize how great may be the value of
language as evidence if we study it in relation to those other
features of culture of which its words are but symbols.   Let us
therefore examine the nomenclature of the two forms of
canoe, to see whether it throws any light on our problem.

If we examine the names of the canoes, and of different
parts of the canoe in Oceania, we find that some have a far
wider distribution than others, and that the word which
has by far the widest is the term for the float of the
outrigger canoe.   Often this word, some form of *sama*, is
combined with some form of *waga* or *vaka* as the term for the
canoe ; but *sama* is often found as the term for the float where
the canoe has quite a different name.   This use of the *sama*
for the float in cases where the canoe itself is differently named
is, as Friederici has pointed out, naturally to be explained if
the outrigger has been adopted by peoples who previously
had only the simple dug-out.   It shows that the outrigger
has been carried widely through Austronesia by a people
who used the word *sama* for the float ; and since we can be
confident that the direction of spread has been from Indonesia
to Polynesia and not *vice versa*, it is evident that, if the outrigger evolved from the double canoe, the evolution must
have taken place either in Indonesia or in a region on the path
of migration where at present we have no evidence of the use
of the double canoe.

The wide distribution of the word makes it highly probable
that if the outrigger has been the outcome of the double
canoe, the evolution has taken place once and once only.   If
the evolution had taken place independently in different

places, it is most unlikely that there would be found the great uniformity in the name of the float, which is so striking a feature of the nomenclature of the Austronesian canoe.

Another term of more importance as evidence is the word *kiato*, which is the almost universal Polynesian term for the booms of the outrigger. This word differs from *sama*, however, in being limited, in its clearly recognizable form, to Polynesia and to islands where relatively recent Polynesian influence can be confidently assumed. If there be a genetic relation between the double canoe and the outrigger, we should not only expect that the outrigger would have the same name as one of the parts of the double canoe, as we have already seen to be the case, but we should also expect the booms to show by their names that they are representative of the structure connecting the two constituents of the double canoe. Friederici gives the word for the connecting timber of the double canoe as *kiato* in Tonga and the Cook Islands, and *iato* in Samoa. The fact that the word *kiato* is used for the connection between the two parts of a double canoe and for that between the body and float of an outrigger canoe, only points to the derivation of one from the other ; it does now show whether the second canoe is an elaboration of a float, or the float a degeneration of the second canoe. The booms and the connection between the two canoes should be homologous structures, to borrow a biological expression ; but the use of a common term for the two structures does not indicate the direction of evolution. It is perhaps easier to understand the persistence of the word if the booms be the degenerate representatives of the more complex structure joining two canoes. Though the evidence is far from being conclusive, it weighs a little on the side of the superiority of the double canoe.

More cogent evidence is derived from the use of the word *kiatu*, which has been recorded by Friederici in the Gambier

Islands. In these islands, the canoe has disappeared and the natives use only a raft, but this raft is called *kiatu*, the word used elsewhere for float and the connecting part of the double canoe. In this case it is quite certain that we have to do with degeneration. There are two possibilities: one, that the raft has been directly derived from the double canoe, the canoes becoming smaller and smaller while the middle connection between the two canoes has grown in size and importance until only this part remains, and has given its name to the whole. The other possibility is that the raft of the Gambier Islands represents rather the outrigger of an outrigger canoe, in which case we again have to do with degeneration. The fact that degeneration is so clearly in evidence in the case of the Polynesian canoe, makes it probable that degeneration has also produced the outrigger canoe.

I have so far considered what can be learned from the distribution and mode of use of the two words *sama* and *kiatu*, and I must consider the nomenclature for other parts of the canoe more briefly. The most prominent fact concerning this nomenclature is that it shows far greater variability than that for the float and booms. Friederici has recorded a large collection of terms for the attachment of the float to the booms, from which it becomes evident that there is great variability in place of the considerable uniformity in the case of the booms, and almost the unanimity in the nomenclature for the float. Corresponding with this diversity in nomenclature, an equally great diversity is found in the nature of the connections. Dr Haddon has distinguished four main types of mode of attachment, and one of these, which he calls the stick attachment, has, he says, no less than six varieties. The question before us is whether this variety in form and name follows most naturally from the priority of the double canoe or of the outrigger.

The importance of this diversity is that it points to the

presence of some factor or factors leading to modification of the attachment between booms and float which has taken place independently in many different places, as distinguished from the single evolution which is indicated by the uniformity in the name for the float. Let us first inquire whether there is any feature of the evolution of the outrigger from the double canoe that would lead to variability in form and a name of the attachment between float and booms. It is evident that if one element of a double canoe degenerated into a float, there would come into existence a space between booms and float that would have to be filled, and this would provide a motive for indirect attachment. If, however, this evolution took place in one region only, as is indicated by the wide distribution of the word *sama* for float, we should expect uniformity in place of the great diversity that actually exists. It becomes improbable that the different forms of indirect attachment are to be explained directly by the process of degeneration of the canoe into a float.

If the diversity in name and form of this attachment be thus taken in conjunction with the uniformity in the nomenclature for the float, it is not possible to ascribe the diversity to the process of derivation of the float from a canoe, which might seem at first sight to afford its most natural explanation. Let us, therefore, inquire whether it is possible to explain this diversity by any factor which would come into existence after the outrigger canoe had become a fully developed structure. One such factor can be distinguished. There is no doubt that in many places the dug-out canoe with outrigger has had its sides raised by the addition of boards which, following Dr Haddon, I shall call wash-strakes. This would make necessary some modification of the attachment of the booms, save in the exceptional cases in which the booms pierce the sides of the canoe. One result of the addition of the wash-strakes will be to raise the ends of the booms far above the water, and the stick and other forms of attachment may come into use as a means of connecting the float with the booms thus separated from it. This is a process which may have taken place independently in many different places, thus accounting for the diversity in name of the attachment. A feature of structure and nomenclature that would seem at first sight to be most naturally explained by the evolution of the outrigger from the double canoe is found on closer consideration to be more naturally explained as the result of a process which occurred independently in many places after the outrigger canoe had come into being. This mode of studying the problem leaves us still with the problem unsolved, for the demonstration that the attachment between booms and float has undergone independent development in many places still leaves us with its origin undetermined.

I have so far considered only the single outrigger canoe. If this form of canoe has been derived from the double canoe, the possibility suggests itself that the double outrigger may have been derived from a triple canoe, the two outer elements of the triple structure degenerating into floats. If this process could be shown to have occurred, it would increase the probability in favour of the single outrigger from the double canoe. We do not know of any case in which the triple canoe is as well established an institution as the double form, but three canoes lashed together are used by the Motu in their annual trading migration to the Papuan Gulf. Sometimes more than three canoes are lashed together for the outward journey, and the number is always increased for the return journey. While there is thus no great degree of definiteness in the existing number of canoes out of which the composite structures are made, it is noteworthy that no matter of how many elements these canoes are formed, they are always called *lakatoi*, a word which means " three canoes," and the established character of this word points to the triple canoe as a definite feature of Motu culture. The existence of the triple canoe, and at no great distance from one centre of distribution of the double outrigger, may be accepted as a fact.

An alternative explanation of the double outrigger is that it has arisen from the single form by a process of addition, but we have at present too little evidence to allow any conclusion. The origin from the triple canoe cannot be held to be more than a conjecture to stimulate us to look for other evidence of the former presence of the triple canoe elsewhere.

The outrigger canoe, both in its single and double forms, presents many other features of interest and raises several problems. I must be content, however, with this review of the facts in so far as they bear on the possible derivation from double or triple canoes. It will be clear that the evidence is not yet sufficient to allow any positive conclusion. My object in bringing forward the subject is to draw attention to the kind of evidence by means of which we may hope to reach a decision. Any theory of the origin of the outrigger canoe has to explain not only the general features of this form of vessel, but it must also serve to explain its details of structure, distribution and nomenclature.

VIII

SUN-CULT AND MEGALITHS IN OCEANIA [1]

THERE is at present no decisive evidence that the sun was the object of a public religious cult in any part of Polynesia. Roggeveen and his companions [2] observed the inhabitants of Easter island prostrating themselves towards the rising sun, but as these prostrations seem to have had some relation to the stone statues of the island, it would be dangerous to conclude that the sun was the object towards which the prostrations were directed.

Similarly, Gill [3] speaks of an " ancient solar cult " in Mangaia, but it is doubtful whether this is more than an inference from the mode of orientation of the dead.' It probably arises directly out of the belief in the direction of the home of the dead and only corresponds with the direction of the sun if this home lie either east or west. [4]

While there is thus no direct evidence of any cult of the sun in Polynesia, there are features of the ritual of the Areoi organization of eastern Polynesia which point to its essential purpose having been closely associated with the sun.

The Areois were outwardly bands of strolling players and chartered libertines who are best known to ethnologists

[1] Reprinted from the *American Anthropologist*, vol. 17, No. 3, July-Sept., 1915.
[2] See Behrens, *Reise durch die Süd-Lander und um die Welt*, 1737, Leipzig, p. 83 (translated as an Appendix to " Voyage of Captain Don Felipe Gonzalez," *Hakluyt Soc.*, Second series, No. 13, Cambridge, 1908, p. 133 ; for another account, see *The World Displayed*, London, 1773, vol. ix, p. 120).
[3] *Life in the Southern Isles*, London, 1876, p. 75.
[4] Cf. W. J. Perry, *Journal of the Royal Anthropological Institute*, 1914, xliv, 281.

through their practice of infanticide, it being a condition of entrance into the society that with certain exceptions no child of a member should be allowed to survive its birth. This practice of infanticide and the licentious character of the festivals have attracted the attention of those who have described the societies to such a degree that with one exception they have neglected or overlooked the beliefs and practices which evidently formed the essential purpose of the societies. There can be little doubt that the features which have hitherto attracted so much attention are only superficial, perhaps only recent, additions to a ritual which had a deep and truly religious origin.

The practice of infanticide was confined to the Areois of the Society Islands and seems to have been wholly absent in other groups such as the Marquesas. Even in Tahiti it was probably a late growth, a special development of the practice of infanticide as it existed widely throughout Polynesia.[1] Similarly, the licentious dances and representations of the Areois were limited to the lowest rank of the societies and seem even among them to have been only a fair sample of the morals of the people as a whole.[2]

In seeking for the deeper meaning of the societies, the first point to note is the resemblance to the secret organizations found in other parts of Oceania. Each Areoi society contained seven ranks or grades, and the processes of initiation into the society and of raising in rank[3] were of a kind closely similar to those of the secret societies of Melanesia. The first object of this paper is to show that this resemblance is more than superficial and proceeds from a fundamental similarity in the purpose and ritual of the different organizations.

---

[1] See Moerenhout, *Voyages aux îles du grand Océan*, Paris, 1837, i, 500.
[2] Moerenhout, *op. cit.*, i, 498.
[3] Moerenhout, *op. cit.*, p. 491 ; Ellis, *Polynesian Researches*, i, 211 *et seq.*

In Tahiti, whence most of our accounts of the Areois have come, the festive proceedings of the societies were almost continuous, and no features of the ritual have come down to us which give any indication of a deeper meaning. In the Marquesas and some of the Society Islands, however, the active life of the Areois was limited to a portion of the year, and it is this limitation which shows the true meaning of the ritual.[1] In the Marquesas, the Areois were inactive during the season of the year when the sun was north of the equator and came out of their retirement in October to celebrate by means of a festival the return of Mahui,[2] the god who brings fertility and abundance, and is, according to Moerenhout, a personification of the sun. About the time of the southern solstice in December there was a second festival, the chief feature of which was the offering of first-fruits to Mahui. The activity of the Areois came to an end in April or May, the exact date varying with the locality and climate. At this time the god was believed to go to Po, the obscure and dark home of the dead, and the members betook themselves to their *marae* or sacred enclosures to pray for the return of the god from this land of obscurity to Rohoutou noanoa, the home of light and life and the proper abode of the gods. From this time until the following October the Areois were in retreat ; they suspended all their amusements and bemoaned the absence of the god until the time came to celebrate his return at the following equinox. There can be little question that we have here a ritual celebration of the annual death of the sun and of its coming to life again to bring abundance and fertility. The Areois of the Gambier Islands had festivals at the equinoxes in October and April which show that the

[1] Moerenhout, *op. cit.*, pp. 501-2.
[2] The connection of Mahui with the Maui of other parts of Polynesia is doubtful, but their identification is supported by many features of the history of Maui which suggest the personification of the sun.

societies must have had a purpose and meaning similar to those of the Marquesans.[1]

There can be little doubt that the celebration of the sun must once also have been the purpose of the Areois of Tahiti. The place of the Marquesan god Mahui is taken in Tahiti by Oro, and, though it is only in some of the Society Islands that the celebrations of the Areois had any seasonal character, it is probable that Oro was also a sun-god, and that it is only by the exaggeration of the pleasure-seeking aspect of the societies and the accretion of the practice of infanticide that the true ritual has been obscured.

If now we turn to the secret societies of Melanesia, we find evidence pointing clearly to the seasonal character of their celebrations and to the possibility that they represent the annual birth and death of the sun. Just as it is the external and obvious features of the Areoi societies which have absorbed the attention of ethnologists in the eastern Pacific, so is it certain obvious and external features which have almost exclusively attracted them in New Britain. We have abundant accounts of the dances and masks, and of the functions of the societies as associations by means of which one section of the community acquires wealth by terrorization and blackmail, but among all the accounts I have only found one to record a feature which furnishes the clue to the deeper meaning of these societies. The Rev. R. H. Rickard tells us [2] that the Dukduk, which is one of the two chief objects of the ritual of the society, dies annually at one season of the year and comes to life again at another. We have here an annual representation of the birth, life, and death of some mysterious being. We know of nothing in the ritual of these societies which points to the sun as the being so represented. We have only the seasonal character of the celebration, and when we

[1] Moerenhout, i, 110.
[2] *Proc. Roy. Soc. Victoria*, 1891, iii, 75.

examine this in detail we find that it differs from the annual celebration of the Marquesas in that the death of the Dukduk takes place at the beginning of the north-west monsoon and the new birth at its end, the period of activity of the Dukduk thus corresponding approximately with that of the retirement of the Areois.

While there is thus no direct evidence that the function of the Dukduk societies is to celebrate the annual birth and death of the sun, there is evidence of rites connected with the sun in a neighbouring part of New Britain.

In one district of the island of Vuatom, in the island of Vurar, and at one place on the mainland of New Britain, a festival takes place when the sun has reached the southern limit of its course.[1] In this festival, which lasts for three days, offerings of the fruits of the earth are made to the sun, and rites are performed which are believed to keep the sun in its proper course. It is clear that it is the annual course of the sun which determines the performance of the rites, for this takes place at the time when the sun reaches its southernmost point as determined by its position in relation to certain hills. The offerings of food which appear to be firstfruits also point to a close resemblance with the leading motive of the celebrations of the Areoi. On the other hand, the rites of Vuatom have features such as the rigorous exclusion of women and the plundering of gardens which form points of resemblance with Melanesian secret societies.

The people of the district where the sun is thus celebrated have certain characteristics of language which show them to be distinct from their neighbours. It would seem as if they practise, as part of their general religious cult, a rite which in neighbouring regions of New Britain has become part of a secret ritual.

---

[1] O. Meyer, *Anthropos*, 1908, iii, 700 and J. Meier, *Anthropos*, 1912, viii, 706.

We have evidence of the importance of the sun in the religion of another part of the Bismarck Archipelago. In the more northern parts of New Ireland, an object called *oara* is made to represent the sun rising out of the sea, and at the end of the rites this object is burnt together with the skull of a dead man which has been dug up soon after interment.[1] It is probably more than a coincidence that the masks of the Dukduk should also be burnt on the day when the annual death of this being is celebrated.

The evidence that the celebration of the birth, life, and death of the Dukduk represents the annual changes of the sun is thus indirect and conjectural. It will become more probable, however, if it is possible to find any connection with the sun in the ritual of the secret societies of other parts of Melanesia. Passing southward, societies called Rukruk, similar to the Dukduk of New Britain, exist in northern Bougainville. We know very little about their customs, but one obvious feature is the wearing of peculiar head-dresses which often have a globular form. In the south of Bougainville, the sun forms a prominent object in decorative art.[2]

In the British Solomon Islands, secret societies called Matambala formerly existed in Florida, and here we have definite evidence of the seasonal character of the celebrations.[3] They began in the month when the canarium-nuts ripen, which form one of the staple foods of the people, and the gathering of nuts to be offered as firstfruits formed the opening rite in the ceremonial. At the end of the proceedings, which seem to have lasted for several months, the masks were burnt as in the Dukduk ceremonies of New Britain. In the course of the celebrations, houses were built so sacred that it is said

[1] Krämer-Bannow, *Zeit. d. Gesell. f. Erdkunde*, Berlin, 1911, p. 21.
[2] Thurnwald, *Forschungen auf den Salomo-Inseln u. d. Bismarck-Archipel*, Berlin, 1912, Bd. i, Tafel xii; also *Ethnopsychologische Studien an Südseevölkern*, Leipzig, 1913, Tafel xxi.
[3] Codrington, *The Melanesians*, 1891, p. 95; also Ray, *Zeitsch. f. afrikan, u. ozean. Sprachen*, 1897, iii, 214.

not even men might enter them, and among the objects which these houses contained were images of the sun and moon.

While there is thus evidence that the sun was an object of importance in the ritual of the Matambala societies, we have no direct evidence that their purpose was to celebrate the annual course of the sun. Indeed, the fact that the ceremonies only took place at intervals of several years shows that, if the annual celebration of the course of the sun was once the object of the rites, they had departed very widely from their original purpose.

Another region of Melanesia which is characterized by the presence of secret societies is that comprising the Banks and Torres Islands and the northern New Hebrides. Here the rites have no obvious seasonal character, and there is nothing which at first sight raises a suspicion that the ritual had anything to do with the annual course of the sun. Nevertheless, there are features which fit in with such a purpose as soon as the possibility is suggested. The people of Mota in the Banks Islands speak of the birth or death of a *tamate*, the mask or other object which acts as the badge of a Tamate or ghost society. One *tamate* is said to have been born at the door of a *gamal* or club-house, while a rite in which the image of a dragon-fly is burnt after the initiation of a new member into the dragon-fly society is said to represent the death of the *tamate*. These expressions point to the representation of the birth, life, and death of the *tamate* as one of the purposes of the secret ritual, and there are so many points of resemblance with the ritual of the Dukduk of New Britain as to leave little doubt that they are manifestations of one and the same culture. It is thus suggested that the representation of the birth, life, and death of the *tamate* in the Banks Islands may have had its origin in the idea of the representation of the annual birth, life, and death of the sun.

The number of Tamate societies in the Banks Islands is very great, but there is one known as the Tamate liwoa or great Tamate, the leading position of which makes it probable that, if any one of the societies is to be associated with the sun, it would be this. There is one feature of the ritual of the Tamate liwoa which suggests relation with the sun. An important feature of initiation into this society is the alignment from east to west of six stakes by means of which the novice advances as he approaches the spot where the special secret of the society is to be revealed to him. The part of the ritual which we know forms only a small proportion of the whole, and a more complete record may show other features of this kind.

More striking, however, than any correspondence in ritual is a similarity in the traditions of origin of the Tamate liwoa and the Areois of Tahiti. The Polynesian societies are said to have been founded as the result of the visit to earth of the god Oro who married a maiden of the earth named Vairaumati, and tradition connects the origin of Tamate liwoa with a supernatural visitor named Wetmatliwo who married a maiden of high rank in the island of Vanua Lava. A great light which filled the house when this person was shown to his wife's parents, and his final disappearance by sinking into the earth, suggest that Wetmatliwo was a personification of the sun. One point of similarity in detail is that while the Tahitian Oro visited his earthly wife by means of a rainbow, a rainbow was also seen by the maiden of the Banks Islands when Wetmatliwo first appeared in her village.

There are other features of the secret organizations of the Banks Islands which suggest a connection with the sun, but this evidence is so scattered and fragmentary that, if it were not for the obvious connection of the Tamate ritual with that of the Dukduk, no great importance could have been attached to it. It is only the combination of the evidence from the secret rituals of New Britain, the Solomon, and Banks Islands which enables us to conclude that one of the purposes of this ritual was the celebration of the annual course of the sun by the anthropomorphic simile of birth and death.

The similarity of the ritual of the secret societies of four different parts of Oceania raises the problem which faces the ethnologist at every turn of his path, whether he has to do with independent origin or with community of culture. In the case before us, the resemblances in detail are so close, and the connection of the cultures of which the secret societies form part so obvious, that I do not suppose there will be any who will venture to put forward the plea of independent origin. The most that could be said from this point of view is that the similarities in belief and practice of the people of the Marquesas and Tahiti, the Banks Islands, the Solomon Islands, and New Britain in this respect are the outcome of some definite idea common to these peoples, not merely as part of the general furniture of the human mind, but through some cultural element common to the different peoples.

I propose, however, to leave such a vague possibility on one side and to assume with confidence that the ideas and practices found in these four parts of Oceania have a common source. The question next to be considered is whether the common source whence the four sets of ideas and practices have been derived is to be placed within or without the limits of Oceania. Are these elements of culture the result of a development which has taken place in some part of Oceania and radiated thence to the places where they are now found, or have they been transported from some other part of the world to the Bismarck Archipelago, the Solomon Islands, southern Melanesia, and eastern Polynesia ? I believe that there is one feature of the beliefs and practices which makes it possible to answer this question.

We have been led by the comparison of the secret societies

of the four regions to conclude that the central idea underlying them is the representation of the annual course of the
sun by means of the anthropomorphic processes of birth and
death. All four regions are in the tropics. New Britain is
only about five and the Marquesas and the Solomons only
about ten to twelve degrees south of the Equator ; such
annual movements of the sun as take place in these regions
would not be likely to suggest the birth and death of a human
being or of an anthropomorphic god. The annual movements
of the sun in the equatorial belt are associated with change
in the prevailing direction of the wind and in the amount of
the rainfall, and consequently with the luxuriance of vegetation, but the changes in the luminosity and heat-giving power
of the sun are not sufficiently great to suggest a simile with
birth and death. Nor does it seem likely that the annual
changes in the position of the sun would have become the
sign for the practices of special religious rites unless there had
been some extraneous source which would have led the people
to attend to these changes and charged them with such
emotional tone as to make them the motive for religious rites.
The representation of the sun's annual movements by the
events of birth and death becomes much more easy to understand if the idea were brought to these tropical regions from
a latitude where the representation would have a real meaning
and be concordant with the behaviour of the sun.

If, then, the central idea underlying the ritual of the Areoi,
Dukduk, Matambala, and Tamate societies be the representation of the sun's movements by the simile of birth, life, and
death, we are driven to the view that the idea and the result-
ing cult must have been introduced into Oceania by a people
who came from some latitude where the simile would have a
meaning. There can be little question that such a latitude
must be placed in the northern hemisphere for, if we except
the southern part of South America and perhaps the south of

New Zealand, there is no part of the southern hemisphere which could have been the home of such an idea.

This cult of the sun forms part of a secret ritual confined to men and associated in at least three of the four places with a cult of dead ancestors. I show elsewhere [1] that the secret cults of Melanesia embody in a more or less pure form the religious practices of an immigrant people. I do not here propose to consider the evidence for this. I must be content to point out that the considerations now brought forward only serve to confirm a conclusion reached by the general study of the secret organizations of Melanesia.

The conclusion so far reached is that the secret rituals of Oceania which have the sun as their object belong to an immigrant culture which has come from a widely distant part of the world. I have now to consider whether it is possible that this same people may also have been the architects of the stone buildings and images which form so great a mystery of the islands of the Pacific.

Here again I will begin with eastern Polynesia. The Areoi societies held their celebrations in an enclosure called *marae* or *marai* at one end of which was situated a pyramidal structure with steps leading to a platform on which were placed the images of the gods during the religious celebrations of the people. The *marae* was used for religious ceremonial unconnected with the Areoi societies, but there seems to be no doubt that the Areois were particularly associated with it. In the pyramid of the *marae*, we have one of the best examples of the megalithic architecture of Polynesia. One such pyramid in the western part of the island of Tahiti was 267 feet in length and 87 feet in breadth at the base. All were built of large stones without cement, but so carefully shaped that they fitted together closely and formed durable structures.[2]

---

[1] *The History of Melanesian Society*, Cambridge, 1914.
[2] Captain Cook's *Journal*, London, 1893, p. 83.

In the Marquesas, another home of the Areois, there were similarly constructed platforms of a hundred yards in length, and many of the shaped and closely-fitting blocks of which these structures were composed were as many as eight feet in length.[1] On these platforms were pyramidal " altars " and they were surrounded by enormous upright stones.[2] This association of the distribution of the Areois with the presence of megalithic structures suggests that the immigrants to whom I have ascribed the cult of the sun may also have been the people who introduced the art of building the stone structures which have so greatly excited the wonder of visitors to Polynesia.

It is in the Caroline Islands that these stone structures have reached their acme in size and complexity. If there be anything in my hypothesis, we should expect to find manifestations of the religious ideas of those who founded the Areoi societies here also. Nor are they lacking. In the Marianne or Ladrone Islands there were associations of persons which suggest an intermediate condition between the Areois of Tahiti and the occupants of the club-house of Melanesia.[3] We know very little about these associations, but their relation to the Areois of the east is clearly shown by the name they bore, Urritois or Ulitaos, which is merely another form of the Tahitian word, Areoi, the latter word having suffered the elision of a consonant, as so frequently occurs in Polynesia. Similar associations flourished in the Carolines, and, though we know still less of them than of the Urritois of the Ladrones, we can be confident that they had a similar character. Societies very closely related to the Areois thus existed in

---

[1] Porter, *Journal of a Cruise Made to the Pacific Ocean*, New York, 1822, ii, 38.

[2] Clavel, *Les Marquisiens*, Paris, 1885, p. 69.

[3] Le Gobien, *Histoires des Iles Marianes*, Paris, 1770, p. 203 ; Freycinct, *Voyage autour du Monde*, 1829, ii, 368, 370 ; Meinicke, *Die Inseln des stillen Oceans*, 1876, ii, 407.

this region in conjunction with stone structures similar to those of eastern Polynesia.

There is a remarkable point of similarity between the traditions concerning the origins of these stone structures and of the Areoi societies of Tahiti. The ruins of Nan-matal on the east coast of Ponape in the Carolines are reputed to have been built by two brothers, Olochipa and Olochopa.[1] In the tradition of the foundation of the Areois of Tahiti, a very prominent part was taken by two brothers Orotetefa and Urutetefa.[2] The interchanges between *r* and *l*, *t* and *ch* and *p* and *f* are so frequent in Oceania as to suggest that these two pairs of names are variants of one original, so that we have in the traditions of these two groups of islands nearly four thousand miles apart, a most striking similarity of the names of pairs of brothers to whom prominent features of the culture are ascribed. In one case the brothers founded societies whose aim it was to celebrate the annual changes of the sun, while rude stone buildings were the handiwork of the others.

A recent account by Hambruch[3] shows that the resemblance between the Ponape and Tahiti names is not quite as close as would appear from previous records. Hambruch calls the two founders of the stone buildings, Sipe and Saupa, but against this he states that the place, Matolenim, where the structures were built, was formerly called *sau nalan* which means " the sun."

Though the resemblance in the names of the two culture heroes of Ponape and Tahiti is not as close as once seemed to be the case, it cannot be neglected. It may be that the two words have some meaning which would reduce the importance of the similarity, but taken in conjunction with the close

[1] Christian, *Caroline Islands*, London, 1899, p. 81.
[2] Ellis, *Polynesian Researches*, 1829, i, 311 ; Moerenhout, *op. cit.*, i, 487.
[3] Korr, *Bl. f. Anth., Ethnol. u. Urgesch.*, 1911, xlii, 121.

resemblance of the names of the societies in the two places, it affords striking corroborative evidence supporting the conclusion suggested by the distribution of societies and monuments, that both are the work of one people.

If the stone monuments and secret societies of Polynesia have had a common source, we should expect to find an association between the two elements of culture in Melanesia, and this is so. We know of stone structures in several parts of Melanesia, viz., the northern New Hebrides, Santa Maria in the Banks Islands, Loh in the Torres Islands, Ysabel in the Solomons, and Fiji.[1] The Banks and Torres Islands and the northern New Hebrides are strongholds of the secret cults, and though the only island in the Solomons in which we know of the existence of secret societies is Florida, there is a definite tradition that this society came to Florida from Ysabel. The distribution of stone structures in Melanesia is just as it should be if the ghost societies and the stone buildings were the work of one and the same people.

The evidence for the connection of stone structures with secret societies is even more definite in Fiji. The Nanga societies of Viti Levu take this name from their meeting places, oblong enclosures, consisting of two or more compartments, surrounded by stone walls.[2] The resemblance of these enclosures to the *marae* of Polynesia has struck more than one observer and the similarity extends to detail. At one end of each main compartment of the *nanga* there were truncated pyramids which served as platforms, evidently representatives of the pyramids of the *marae* of Tahiti measured by Captain Cook. Further, both *marae* and *nanga* were oriented with their long axes east and west, though the two differ in that the

---

[1] See *History of Melanesian Society*, vol. ii, p. 427.
[2] L. Fison, *Journ. Anth. Inst.*, 1885, xiv, 14 ; Joske, *Internat Arch. f. Ethnog.*, 1889, ii, 254 ; B. Thomson, *The Fijians*, 1908, p. 147

pyramids were at the western end of the *marae* [1] and at the eastern end of the *nanga*. [2]

There is thus a remarkable correspondence between the distribution of stone structures and secret societies in Oceania which points strongly, if not yet decisively, to the introducers of the secret cult of the sun having been the architects of the stone buildings which form one of the chief mysteries of the islands of the Pacific.

It is even possible that we may have here the clue to the greatest mystery of all, the great stone statues of Easter Island. There is reason to suppose that these statues are not so unique as is often supposed. According to Moerenhout, [3] similar statues, though not so large, exist in the islands of Pitcairn and Laivaivai; he believes that such colossal figures once existed in many other islands, but have been destroyed or have fallen into ruins. In the Marquesas and Society Islands, likewise, stone figures in human form have been found which resemble those of the smaller and more eastward islands enough to suggest a common origin. Moerenhout believes that such stone figures and statues had a common meaning and were all representatives of beings called *tii* whose function it was to mark the limits of the sea and land, to maintain harmony between the two elements and prevent their encroachment upon one another. I venture, though very diffidently, to extend the comparison. At one end of a club-house of Santa Maria in the Banks Islands, there are ancient stone figures which, in one respect at least, resemble the colossal statues of Easter Island. In each instance the head is covered. This head-covering is very frequent in one variety of the representations of the human figure found throughout Melanesia, and is almost certainly connected with

---

[1] Captain Cook's *Journal*, 1893, p. 83.
[2] A further point of resemblance between the *marae* and *nanga* is that both were the scene of offerings of firstfruits.
[3] *Op. cit.*, i, 461. See p. 222.

the importance of head-coverings in the ritual of the secret societies. It is therefore of interest that a head-covering should be a prominent feature of the statues of Easter Island. Such a point of resemblance, standing alone, would have little significance, but taken in conjunction with the other correspondences and similarities pointed out in this essay, we must not ignore the possibility that we may have here only another expression of the art of the people I suppose to have introduced the cult of the sun into Oceania.

I cannot consider here how far it is possible to connect the stone-work and sun-cult of Oceania with the megalithic monuments and sun-cults of other parts of the world. Megalithic monuments elsewhere are associated with a cult of the sun, and the occurrence of this association in the islands of the Pacific Ocean must serve to strengthen the position of those who hold that the art of.building megalithic monuments has spread from one source. I must be content here to mention certain megalithic monuments of Polynesia which raise a difficulty.

The island of the Pacific which holds examples of megalithic structures most closely resembling those of other parts of the world is Tongatabu, where there are trilithic monuments so like those of Europe that the idea of a common source must rise to the mind of even the most strenuous advocate of independent origin. It is not possible at present to bring these monuments into relation with those of other parts of Oceania by connecting them with a cult of the sun, but Hambruch tells us that tradition points to the builders of the stone work of Ponape as having come from Tonga. It may be that Tongatabu forms the intermediate link between the stone-work of the Carolines and the megalithic monuments of other parts of the world.

I have dealt elsewhere [1] with the relation between these

[1] *History of Melanesian Society*, vol. ii, p. 549.

Tongan monuments and the pyramids of other parts of Oceania, and have suggested that these two ancient forms of monument may be expressions of the ideas of two different streams of the megalithic culture. I cannot deal with this matter here ; to do so would take me far beyond the relation of sun-cult and megaliths, which is the subject of this essay.

IX

THE PEOPLING OF POLYNESIA [1]

FEW subjects connected with the history of Mankind have excited a greater sense of wonder and mystery than the peopling of the islands of the Pacific Ocean. It has seemed hardly possible that islands, so widely scattered over so vast a sea, could have been occupied with the means of navigation which it would seem at first sight natural to ascribe to early man. Especially difficult has it been to account for the great images and monuments of stone, the construction of which seems far beyond the powers of such people as we now know in the Pacific Isles. Some have even been led to think that the Polynesians represent the people of an ancient continent, whose mountain-tops formed the bases to islands, and groups of islands which are now all that is left above the surface of the sea. The explanation of Polynesian culture which is now widely current goes to the opposite extreme, and assumes that the peopling of Polynesia is quite recent. It is accepted by most of those who have studied Polynesian culture on the spot, and I hope it will not be thought presumptuous if one who only knows the outskirts of Polynesian culture, and that superficially, takes the opportunity of looking at the subject afresh from the standpoint of the science of ethnology.

Let us first inquire what are the grounds for the belief in the comparative modernity of Polynesian culture. I begin with one which I believe to have had a great influence among

---

[1] Address delivered in New Zealand, 1914.

ethnologists in general, though I do not know that it has been explicitly put forward as an argument by special students of Polynesian lore. This reason is the great uniformity of Polynesian languages. Nowhere else in the world do we find such uniformity spread over so large an area ; nowhere else do we find peoples separated so widely, and having so little communication with one another. Yet their languages are so akin that in a day or two the stranger can make use of the native tongue for all ordinary purposes of daily intercourse. It is generally supposed that living creatures have only to be separated and isolated from one another, and changes arise, which, in the case of animals and plants, give rise to forms regarded as distinct species. If this law, which seems to hold good of plants and animals, be also applied to man and his culture, we should expect to find diversity in speech, one of the most mobile of man's activities. Biology and human variety elsewhere lead us to suppose that the unity of Polynesian language is the result of recent dispersal from some common centre.

When, further, this biological consideration is found to be supported by the traditions of the people themselves, there is small reason for surprise that the peopling of Polynesia within recent times should have become with many almost a settled article of faith.

But even on superficial considerations there are some difficulties which may be noticed at the outset.

The evidence for recent origin is derived largely from the traditions and pedigrees of the Polynesians. Not only is there an extraordinary correspondence in the traditions of origin of the people in many different parts of the Pacific, but there is also a close agreement in the details of pedigrees preserved by Maori, Rarotongan and Tahitian, and by Tahitian and Hawaiian. Moreover, their pedigrees allow us to assign a date to the divergence of the peoples from one another, which approximately dates about 700 years ago.

There is universal agreement that the ancestors of the Polynesians reached the Pacific by way of the Malay Archipelago,
but 700, or even 1000 years ago bring us within historical
times, and it is most unlikely that any great movement of
such a people as the Polynesians through this archipelago
could have taken place at so recent a date. One way of
escaping this difficulty is that the dispersion at this time took
place from some centre—probably the Samoan and Tongan
groups, and that the settlement of this centre had taken
place long before. Samoan traditions gives us evidence of
such a process. Let us accept this position and inquire
whether all our difficulties are thus removed.

First, may be mentioned the stone images of such places
as Easter and Pitcairn Islands. These images are so unlike
anything now made by the people of Polynesia ; they show
the presence of a culture so dissimilar from that of the present
time, that it is difficult to believe that they can only have
been made seven hundred years ago. The complete loss of
the knowledge of the monuments might be accepted if it had
occurred in Melanesia or Central Africa, but it is difficult to
understand that a people who have borne in their minds the
minute details of ancestry and migration for seven hundred
years, should have wholly forgotten the building and even
the meaning of these monuments if they are contemporaneous.
The student of Polynesia is like any other man, he cannot eat
his cake and have it too. If the memory of the Polynesian
be so good in one direction, it cannot be so untrustworthy in
another. His loss of knowledge of the monuments of Easter
Island points to an antiquity far greater than that of the
ancestors and migrations the memory of which has been so
accurately preserved. Easter and Pitcairn Islands lie at the
furthest eastern limits of Polynesia. If they were inhabited
previous to a migration from Samoa and its neighbourhood
seven hundred years ago, it will be impossible to postulate

the absence of early population also from the far larger and more accessible islands which lie between Samoa and Easter Islands.

Before I leave this subject I must raise a question. Why should these monuments now be found only in such remote and tiny islands as Easter and Pitcairn ? I venture to answer that it is owing to their remoteness and small size that they have escaped later influences which have led to the destruction of similar monuments elsewhere. It is noteworthy that Moerenhout,[1] one of our best authorities, states that such monuments as those of Easter Island were once to be found far more widely in the Pacific Islands.

So far, I have been content to raise one or two difficulties which face the believer in the recent arrival of Polynesian culture. I shall now proceed to examine some elements of this culture in more detail and inquire how the matter stands in the light of our present knowledge of human culture in general.

The first point to be considered is whether Polynesian culture is simple or complex. To the older ethnologist, there is nothing exceptional in the belief that Polynesian culture is simple, and has been the outcome of the development of beliefs and practices brought by one people to the Pacific. The modern trend in ethnology, though far from being accepted by all, is to regard human culture as the result of a vast complexity produced through the superposition of a series of cultures one above another. It is supposed that there have taken place at long intervals of time, and for reasons at present little understood,[2] a series of wide dispersals of mankind over the world. We know that movements of mankind such as would be produced by such dispersals have taken place in Europe and Asia, not only within historical times, but in the long ages which preceded them. Even if

[1] *Voyages aux îles du grand Océan*, Paris, 1837.
[2] But see p. 171.

Q

we go back to the palæolithic age of Europe, perhaps twenty thousand years ago, we find evidence of just such movements of peoples as have taken place in historical times. That European and Asiatic cultures, and in less measure those of Africa, are highly complex is certain, and the same is true of the cultures of Indonesia and Melanesia. The parts of the world where this complexity is not universally accepted are Australia, Polynesia and America.

The most strenuous advocate of complexity must acknowledge that Polynesia presents peculiar conditions which make simplicity possible. In addition to the uniformity of language already considered, it may be pointed out that its scattered islands can only be reached by skilled navigators; and this suggests that the peopling of these islands only became possible at a relatively late stage of human development, so that the wave on wave of culture which have reached other parts of the world have not acted upon this region. On the other hand, two considerations must be mentioned: one, that there is much reason to believe that Asia has been one of the chief centres from which the dispersions of varieties of human culture has taken place, and Polynesia is not remote from Asia; and secondly, that some of the migrations by which the complexity of culture in general has been produced, and notably that which carried the art of building great monuments of stone, have almost certainly travelled by sea.

The simplicity or complexity of Polynesian culture cannot be settled, however, by *a priori* considerations. It is only by the examination and analysis of Polynesian culture itself and by comparing it with other cultures that the solution can be found. I propose to consider briefly certain features of Polynesian culture, leaving on one side for a time the culture of New Zealand.

In the endeavour to ascertain whether a culture is simple or complex, it is usually necessary to study it, not by itself, but in relation to other cultures with which it is connected. I will begin, therefore, by briefly considering the known cultural affinities of Polynesia, and for this purpose I will take that element of culture which has already formed the chief object of attention among students, the language of Polynesia. Consider, first, the situation of Polynesia. It lies in direct geographical continuity with America on one side, and with Australia, Melanesia, the Malay Archipelago and the continent of Asia on the other. If now we compare the languages of Polynesia with those of these other areas, we find only the most remote resemblances with those of America, such resemblances as may be nothing more than the accidental similarities such as we may expect to find in any large collection of facts. Next, it is found that there is no relation with the languages of Australia, and with certain exceptions to which I shall come shortly, with Chinese or with other languages of the continent of Asia.

It is far otherwise when we turn to Melanesia, whose highly diversified languages have much in common· with those of Polynesia in phonetic character, in grammatical structure, and in vocabulary. The relation between the two groups of languages is exactly such as might be expected if the people or peoples who have settled in Polynesia blended in Melanesia with an aboriginal population which spoke a vast variety of tongues. The view which explains the facts most satisfactorily is that the islands of Melanesia were once occupied by a number of peoples differing from one another in speech, among whom there came a unifying agent or agents, a branch or branches of the same people or peoples who, further afield, became the ancestors of the Polynesians.

If now we proceed westwards we find another relative of Polynesian speech in the languages of the Malay Archipelago, languages generally classed together under the title of Indonesian. The connection has recently been denied by

Churchill,[1] but it is one that we can accept with confidence. The connection is such as might be expected if the peoples I have supposed to have settled in Melanesia and Polynesia came by way of the Malay Archipelago. The linguistic similarities do not stop, however, with this archipelago, but extend to the continent of Asia, the connection being especially with the languages of south-eastern Asia known as the Mon-Khmer languages, while other allies are found in Assam, Mon-Khmer and India, the languages of such people as the Mundas and Santhals bearing a definite affinity with those of the Pacific Islands.

The discovery of these wide affinities is due to Father Schmidt, who has classed together the languages of Polynesia, Melanesia and Indonesia as Austronesian, and those of the Mon-Khmer and Munda peoples as Austro-Asiatic. It is a favourite occupation of students of Polynesian culture to trace the derivation of Polynesian words from Sanscrit. If we are to use language as our guide, the representatives of Maori or Tahitian are not to be found in the composers of the Vedic hymns, the proud introducers of Aryan culture into India, but among wild jungle peoples such as the Santhals or Mundas. If language is to be our guide, and if we assume the physical and cultural unity of the Polynesian peoples, it is the Santhal or Munda that we must accept as the Indian representatives of Maori or Tahitian. If, on the other hand, we are prepared to accept the complexity of Polynesian culture, it may be possible to discover other ways of accounting for the affinities in language between the two sets of people.

Let us now return to Melanesia, which in spite of the difference of its inhabitants in physical character, furnishes the nearest relative of Polynesian culture. It is impossible here to consider in more than the briefest outline the many

---

[1] *Easter Island and the Rapanui Speech and the Peopling of south-east Polynesia*, 1912.

points of resemblance in culture between the two peoples, and I shall have to confine my attention to one element of culture, the modes of treating the bodies of the dead. I will begin by considering those found in Polynesia itself.

A frequent mode of disposal is interment, and of this there are two distinct varieties : one, in which the body is buried in the sitting position with the limbs tightly bound ; the other, in which the body is bound in the extended position, sometimes within the house. Where this method is especially in vogue, among the chiefs of Tonga and Samoa that is to say, the body is placed in a vault constructed of stones.

Another mode of treatment is preservation above the ground. In this mode the body is laid in the extended position, either exposed to the sun or definitely embalmed, until it comes to resemble the mummies of other parts of the world. Sometimes the body is laid in a canoe, sometimes on a platform, and in the latter case there is reason to believe that the platform may represent a house. Usually this mode of preservation is only preliminary to the deposition of the skull and other bones in a cave or other secret place, while in other cases, and especially in the island of Mangaia, the body is deposited in a cave from the beginning.

A last mode of treatment is to throw the body into the sea, or send it adrift in a canoe.

Thus, leaving New Zealand out of account, we have no less than five different modes of treating the bodies of the dead : interment in the sitting position ; interment in the extended position in the house or in a vault ; preservation above the ground with mummification and deposition of the bones in a cave or other inaccessible place ; deposition in a cave from the beginning ; and throwing into the sea or casting adrift in a canoe.

There are few customs in which Man is more conservative than in his treatment of the dead. Among ourselves, a new kind of funeral rite, such as cremation, only makes its way very slowly and as the result of strenuous propaganda. Meanwhile, old modes are practised almost untouched, and details of funeral rites persist century after century, even when they are inconvenient, expensive and meaningless to those who practise them. If Polynesian culture is an affair of the last thousand years, we have to suppose either that this variety of funeral rites was brought with them by the early immigrants from their former home, or that these varieties had developed in the relatively simple environment of Polynesia. We can be confident that people will only change their treatment of the dead under the stress of distinct social needs, and it is the duty of those who believe in the simplicity of Polynesian culture to show why there is this variety, and what are the social needs by which it has been produced.

In some cases it is possible to see how varieties of funeral rites may have arisen in Polynesia. Thus, the use of a canoe in many of the funeral rites of Polynesia may be the result of the migration of the people by sea, the canoe being used with the idea of taking back the dead to the home of their fathers, and one mode of disposal, the throwing into the sea or casting adrift in a canoe, may be connected with the same idea. Moreover, disposal in caves is probably only a special manifestation of the set of ideas which lead to the interment in a vault of stones. This mode of interment seems to be only a special mode of preservation ; it was sometimes combined with embalming ; and Mariner [1] saw the dead buried many years before, still well preserved, when the royal vault of Tonga was opened to receive the body of his protector, Finau.

The various modes of disposal found in Polynesia may thus be reduced to two main varieties, interment in the sitting position, and preservation in a cave, in the house, in

[1] *An Account of the Natives of the Tonga Islands*, 1817.

an imitation of a house, or in a vault, which may be regarded as a grave beneath the ground. It is noteworthy that in all these latter forms the body is placed in the extended position, in distinction from the contracted and sitting position in which the bodies of the ordinary people are interred in Melanesia.

If we examine the two main modes of disposal more closely, we find that they are practised by different sections of the population. The use of the extended position, whether in interment or preservation, is especially associated with the chiefs, while interment in the sitting position is practised by ordinary people. There is, though less definitely, a similar association in Melanesia, and this can hardly be due to similarity of conditions, except in so far as there are elements of the population common to those areas. In Melanesia, there is clear evidence that chiefs are representatives of immigrants who came to occupy a special social position wherever they settled, and the similarity of the funeral rites in Polynesia and Melanesia is most naturally to be explained if in Polynesia also the chiefs are the representatives of an immigrant people who believed in the preservation of the dead. I may remark that if this be the case, it would only be an example of a very general rule in human history, a rule which applies among ourselves, since our nobles were originally the descendants of the invading Normans, while the general body of the population are the representatives of the people who inhabited Great Britain before the Norman Conquest.

The two chief varieties of disposal of the dead are not only distinguished by their connection with chiefs and commoners respectively, but also with different ideas concerning the fate of the two classes of the population after death. The commoners interred in the sitting position went to a home, often described as dark and gloomy, which seems to have been located beneath the ground, while the chiefs went at once or after a period of probation, to a home in or near the sky.

Moreover, there is evidence that the two modes of treating the dead were not only associated with different ranks and with different destinations after death, but also with wholly different emotions and sentiments towards the dead. There is clear evidence from certain islands, and especially from Mangaia in the Cook Islands, that the interment in the sitting position was designed to prevent the return of the dead to earth. The binding of the body, and the placing of heavy stones over the grave are said by Gill [1] to have been means to that end. The people thus preventing, as best they could, the return to earth of one section of the population were at the same time keeping among themselves, sometimes even in their houses, the dead of chiefly or royal rank. These two modes of disposal, thus actuated by motives diametrically opposed to one another and practised by different sections of the population, are just such differences as point unmistakably to an origin among different peoples and in widely different surroundings. The continuation of these opposed and contradictory modes of disposal of the dead in Polynesia is just such as might be expected if a people who believed in the preservation of the dead and in their beneficial influence upon the living, settled among a people who feared their dead and removed them as effectually as possible from all contact with the living by putting them below the ground, with every precaution to prevent their return to earth.

Many features of Polynesian culture become explicable by this twofold treatment of the dead. I shall only deal with one of these, the nature of the decorative art. In Polynesia, as in many other parts of the world, there is evidence of the transition, or as it is sometimes called, the degeneration, of

[1] *Life in the Southern Islands*, 1876.

naturalistic designs into geometrical patterns. In Oceania generally, representations of animals or plants or of the human form are found passing in various ways into rectilinear patterns. In Polynesia, the human form thus undergoes change, one of the best examples being that of the Cook-Hervey Islands in which it becomes transformed into the rectilinear pattern characteristic of these islands. Such a process has often been compared with inexactness in copying. Many of us have probably played at a game in which a drawing made by one person is copied by another and the copy again copied by a third, and so on round a circle, until after a time it becomes something wholly different from the picture which began the game. It has been supposed that such transitions as those of the Banks or Cook Islands have arisen in a similar way. There is, however, a most important difference between the two. Where a picture is copied by one person after another, the product is one of which the term degeneration may appropriately be used, the result being usually some meaningless and inartistic object.

The process of the Cook Islands, on the other hand, gives rise to a product which is no whit less artistic or finished, or may be even more artistic and finished than the human representation from which it started. Such a process is not to be explained by carelessness or inexactness, but as the result of blending two forms of artistic expression. It depends either on the introduction of a naturalistic form of design among a people whose art is based upon geometrical patterns, or on the introduction of geometrical designs among a people whose art was of a naturalistic kind. Such a product as the ceremonial adzes of the Cook Islands is best to be explained if a people who had the human figure as the predominant motive of their decorative art, settled among a people with a highly developed form of geometrical art. As the introduced art passed from hand to hand and from generation to generation, a blend took place between the two which resulted in a highly decorative geometrical design, the special form of which has been determined by the human motive with which the examples already shown were so closely related. All that we know of Polynesian and Melanesian art and religion leads us to the view that the transition is to be most readily explained if people who worshipped their ancestors and used representations of their dead in their decorative art, settled among a people who feared the dead and practised a form of art which eschewed all representation of the human form or other natural object, and practised an exclusively geometrical form of decoration. Polynesian art falls into line with the scheme of the twofold nature of Polynesian culture, the later and introduced element of which practised a cult of dead ancestors and kept their dead among themselves as objects to be cherished, if not worshipped.

I propose now to accept this coming into Polynesia of a people who preserved their dead and used the human form as the predominant motive of their decorative art. Let me turn now and inquire whether it is possible to connect this people with other elements of culture that can be linked with people elsewhere. Thus we can bring one element of Polynesian culture into relation with the rest of the world.

The greatest mystery of the Pacific lies in its monuments of stone. If it is possible to assign these monuments to the people who preserved their dead, we shall have gone far towards the solution of one problem of the peopling of Polynesia. We have here a good example of the way in which the study of one area of the world helps us to understand the nature of another. From the study of Polynesia alone, I believe it would be impossible to establish a connection between megalithic monuments and the preservation and cult of the dead. For the evidence showing this connection we have to turn to Melanesia, where we find special organizations, usually classed with secret societies, whose essential motive is a cult of the dead, and there is a remarkable correspondence between the distribution of these societies and the presence of rude stone monuments. Moreover, both monuments and secret cult of the dead are associated with just that practice of preservation and mummification of the dead which we have been led to ascribe to the later element of the population of Polynesia. In Polynesia and Micronesia, we know of organizations resembling those of Melanesia only in two places, in Eastern Polynesia and in the Caroline and Ladrone Islands. It is remarkable that these two places should be the seats of some of the most remarkable of the stone monuments of Oceania. Thus, in Tahiti which seems to have been the chief home of the Areois, we have records of pyramids, as much as two hundred and fifty-seven feet in length, built of large stones without cement. In the Marquesas, where there is reason to believe that the original character of the Areoi organization was preserved with greater fidelity than in Tahiti, platforms are to be found as much as a hundred yards in length, made of blocks of stone as much as eight feet in length, so large as to make it difficult to imagine how they could have been shaped and placed in position by a people whose material culture is now so simple and elementary.

Through these secret organizations we are thus able to connect the megalithic monuments of Polynesia and Melanesia with the cult and preservation of the dead. It remains to inquire whether it is possible to connect the monuments with those of other parts of the world, and thus link the later element of the population of Polynesia with known peoples elsewhere.

We approach here one of the most disputable subjects of archæology. There is so remarkable a similarity in the rude monuments made of large stones all the world over that the idea of their having spread from one source must rise at once to the mind, and where these monuments are

found near to one another and where the surroundings and
paths by which the culture may have travelled are familiar,
it is now widely accepted that megalithic monuments have
arisen in one place and have been distributed thence by the
wanderings of peoples. It is only when similar monuments
are found in places widely remote from our own countries
that this idea of common origin is put on one side, and it is
supposed that the monuments have arisen independently.
The presence of megalithic monuments in places such as the
Polynesian Islands has seemed to many to afford the strongest
argument against their common source. There are many
who are prepared to admit the unity of the monuments of
Europe, Africa, Palestine and India, but whose imagination
will not permit them to extend the journey to the islands of
the Pacific. I may begin by considering one or two points
which make it easier to accept the wide dispersion of a megalithic culture. One is the general distribution of megalithic
monuments near the sea, which makes it most certain that
the megalithic culture travelled by sea. A people who have
travelled from Europe to India and from India to Japan by
sea are just such a people to whom we can safely ascribe that
degree of adventurousness and nautical skill which would
have taken them to Tonga, Easter Island and New Zealand.

Next, it is evident that a people who succeeded in carrying
widely over the world such an art as that of building these
great monuments of stone must have succeeded in implanting
other elements of their culture in their new home. It is
therefore necessary to inquire what are the customs which
we can associate with megaliths elsewhere. There is no doubt
that they are connected with a cult of the dead and with the
preservation of the bodies of the dead.

Moreover, one of the most striking forms taken by the
megalithic art of Polynesia is the pyramid, and the brilliant
work of Elliot Smith has shown the close relation between

the mastaba, the prototype of the Egyptian pyramid, and the dolmen and other forms of megalithic art. We all know how close was the connection between the pyramid of Egypt and the custom of mummification, and it is a fact which cannot but strike the imagination that there should be just this association between the pyramid and mummification in Polynesia. Both pyramid and mummy are crude beside those of Egypt, but this crudeness is only to be expected if they are the distant, perhaps the degenerate relics in remote Pacific isles, of one of the highest cultures which the world has seen. When we consider the absence of metals and the difficulties in the way of even the simplest manufactures, the wonder is that the pyramids of Polynesia should be the imposing monuments they are.

If we reject the view that these monuments and customs of Polynesia have been derived directly or indirectly from those of other parts of the world, we are driven to the alternative explanation by independent origin. We shall have to explain, not only why megaliths and mummies have come into being in Polynesia, but the association between the two likewise. If it were possible to show that there is an essential connection between megaliths and mummies, the advocate of independent origin might have a case, but, in the absence of knowledge of any such connection, the most probable hypothesis is that the two elements of culture exist in combination in the two places because of the common presence of a culture to which they both belonged.

The case for a common origin will become stronger if still other elements of culture can be shown to be common to the two places. Such an element is to be found in the cult of the sun. In Egypt, there is a definite association between the pyramid culture and the sun. Is there evidence of any such connection in Polynesia ? At first sight, it would seem that the question must be answered in the negative.

A superficial survey of the literature of Polynesian culture fails to show any trace of a cult of the sun, but deeper inquiry shows that a cult of the sun was practised by the Areois of Eastern Polynesia, and was probably the main motive of their esoteric rites.[1] This connection between secret rites and the sun-cult is confirmed by the study of Melanesian secret societies. To the association of megaliths and the preservation of the dead common to Polynesia and Egypt, there must also be added the cult of the sun. Here again, there seems to be no essential connection between pyramids, mummification and the sun. The association of the three in these widely separated places is most naturally to be explained if the three elements of culture have come to be associated under the peculiar conditions of some one culture, and have then been carried widely over the world by the wanderings of peoples.

I have now to inquire whether it is possible to trace the route by which this culture travelled. I have already pointed to community of language as an argument for the view that the ancestors of the Polynesians travelled by way of the Malay Archipelago, and there is so much in common between the Polynesians and the inhabitants of the Archipelago that it is by this route that we should expect the megalithic culture to have come. It has been a grave difficulty for the theory of the common origin of Polynesian and other megaliths, that they seem to be absent from this natural path of migration. It is owing to this apparent gap in the distribution of megalithics that Professor Macmillan Brown, who has for long been a strenuous advocate of the common origin of megalithic monuments has been led to suppose that the megalithic culture travelled across the continent of Asia.[2] If, however, it is possible to show that megalithic monuments

---

[1] See p. 223.
[2] *Maori and Polynesian*, 1907.

are present in the Malay Archipelago, this unlikely assumption will no longer be necessary.   The belief that megalithic monuments are absent in the Malay Archipelago is, indeed, without foundation.   Structures closely similar to the dolmens of other parts of the world occur, especially in the island of Sumba in the Eastern part of the archipelago, and Mr Perry has found many other features of belief and ceremony which point to a former wide distribution of the megalithic culture.[1] It must be remembered that some of the best known parts of the archipelago, such as Java, have later become the seats of relatively high cultures with elaborate forms of architecture, and it may even be that here as so often elsewhere, old megalithic monuments have been used to supply the building material of a later age.

It is possible that some of the manifestations of megalithic culture have reached the islands of the Pacific by way of Japan.   Even if this be so, however, it was probably due only to a further extension of a movement which reached Japan by way of the sea.   The elaborate stone buildings of the Caroline Islands may have been one of the resting-places of the megalithic culture from which it radiated northwards to Japan, southwards and eastwards to Tonga and Tahiti. Whatever may have been the path, however, by which the megalithic culture reached Polynesia and Melanesia, there is little doubt that these regions are only outliers of a vast region of distribution, the different parts of which show such geographical continuity, such similarity of meaning and technique, and such correspondence of accompanying features of culture, that by far the most natural explanation is to be found in the wanderings of a single culture, if not of a single people. The later of the two main immigrations out of which the population of Polynesia is composed seem to have been that of a people, probably not far removed from ourselves in

[1] *The Megalithic Culture of Indonesia*, Manchester, 1918.

physical feature and mental character, who, starting from some part of the world still uncertain, have come to form an element common to cultures seemingly so unlike as those of ancient Egypt, the British Isles and Polynesia.   The study of Polynesia suggests that the present movement of one culture widely over the earth which seems to us distinctive of our own era, is but the latest of a series of such movements, of which none stands out as more romantic or more wonderful than the journeys of those whose religious needs led them to erect such vast monuments as the pyramids of Egypt and Tahiti, the trilithons of Nukualofa and Stonehenge.

Of the earliest stratum of the population of Polynesia, I do not propose to speak.   Much in the Maori culture of New Zealand distinguishes it from that of the rest of Polynesia. Though its language is strictly Polynesian in character, it has phonetic features peculiar to it among all the tongues of Polynesia.   Still more important than phonetic difference is the difference of accent, for accent is probably one of the most distinctive and persistent signs of difference of race.

Another feature which in the most striking manner distinguishes New Zealand from the rest of Polynesia is the character of its decorative art.   Everywhere else in Polynesia, the art is either naturalistic or rectilinear, or more usually, as we have already seen, a combination of the two.   Only in New Zealand do we find a pronounced curvilinear art in which the spiral is especially prominent.   Moreover, this curvilinear art is usually combined with the representation of the human form, so that, just as elsewhere in Polynesia, you find transitions between the human form and rectilinear patterns.   The characteristic feature of Maori art is the transition between the human form and spiral or other curvilinear designs.   I have supposed that elsewhere in Polynesia this transition is the result of the settlement of one people with an art devoted especially to the portrayal of the human form among another people with a rectilinear, geometrical art. For New Zealand there are two possibilities. One is, that a people with a curvilinear art settled among a people comparable with the rest of Polynesia, and gave its special character to the art of the earlier population. The alternative is that the megalithic people, with the human figure as the leading motive of their art, found in New Zealand an indigenous population different from that of other parts of Polynesia, because there had settled in New Zealand, but not elsewhere, a people with a curvilinear art who had either failed to reach the rest of Polynesia, or, if they voyaged so far, were so few in number or so poor in influence, that they had no effect upon the culture.

If there is thus in the population of New Zealand an element absent from the rest of Polynesia, we should expect to find some modes of disposing of the bodies of the dead unknown elsewhere, in Polynesia. So there are among the modes of treating the bodies of the dead practised in New Zealand, but almost, if not quite unknown elsewhere in Polynesia, those of placing the corpse in the upright position against a tree, and putting the bones of the dead in a hollow tree-trunk after they have been exposed on a platform.

The evidence thus points to the presence, in New Zealand, of a people who used the spiral and other curvilinear forms in their art and practised a cult in which trees stood in some kind of intimate relation to the dead. Before I consider how these people may have reached New Zealand, and who they can have been, I must mention that there is clear evidence that these people must have found New Zealand already occupied by, or were joined later by, the people who interred their dead in the sitting position. For this mode of burial has been practised not only in New Zealand but also by the Moriori of Chatham Island, its use by this people being alone sufficient to show how ancient the practice is. Its antiquity, however, does not rest on this alone, but is shown by the discovery in excavations of this mode of interment in New Zealand itself, and by the total absence of knowledge on the part of the Maoris of the people who practise this form of funeral rite.

It is evident, therefore, that New Zealand differs from the rest of Polynesia, not in the substitution of one kind of aboriginal inhabitant for another, but in the addition to the aboriginal element of other parts of a third people with a cult of trees and a curvilinear form of art.

I have now to consider who this third people were, and by what route they reached New Zealand. Among other things I have to explain is why they should have failed to reach the rest of Polynesia. I must first point out that the two features of a curvilinear art and a cult of trees are not only absent from, or show but faint signs of their presence, through-out the greater part of Melanesia, but do not appear in any highly developed form until we reach the great island of New Guinea. Moreover, these features are especially developed among the people known as the Massim, who inhabit this island at the south-eastern corner of the island. Traces of them are to be found in the islands of the Bismarck Archipelago and northern part of the Solomons, but on passing southwards are scanty except perhaps in the Santa Cruz Islands, till we come to the southern New Hebrides and New Caledonia.

Beyond all doubt, the south-eastern corner of New Guinea has been a place of much importance in the peopling of the Pacific. Many of the settlers in the islands of Oceania must have coasted the northern shores of New Guinea and have reached, at its south-eastern corner, a parting of the ways, there being here several alternative routes, one eastwards along the southern coast of New Guinea towards Australia ; another northwards towards New Britain and New Ireland ; and still another southwards towards the Solomons. I venture to suggest that still another path has been directly southwards by sea to New Caledonia and avoiding the greater part of

Melanesia, so that New Caledonia would be the point of departure for the still more perilous journey to New Zealand.

Not only would the curvilinear art and the tree cult common to New Guinea and New Zealand be explained thus but also the working of jade or nephrite which is not only common to these places but occurs also in New Caledonia, which I have supposed to be the chief resting-place on the way. The view that there is a culture common to New Guinea and New Zealand has been greatly strengthened by the recent discoveries made on the Kaiserin Augusta River in the German portion of New Guinea. Here, far up the river and evidently the relics of some very old migration, there are preserved heads with marks so closely resembling the tattooing of the Maori that, when combined with other features of culture common to the two peoples, there can be little doubt that the explanation is to be found, not in independent origin, but in the presence of a people and a culture which has passed from one place to the other by the prolongation of a migration from some place still unknown.

I have now briefly sketched a scheme of the peopling of Polynesia and New Zealand. According to this scheme, the population of most parts of Polynesia has two strata to which a third has been added in New Zealand. It only remains to show how this scheme can be brought into harmony with Polynesian traditions. According to these traditions as confirmed by the correspondence of the pedigrees of different islands, the Polynesians reached their present home during the last seven or eight hundred years. It is a general rule in human tradition that it is the recent which especially attracts attention. Compare the wealth of our knowledge of the Norman Conquest with our scanty and uncertain evidence of previous history, still more with our knowledge of Saxon or Roman conditions, or of the many invasions and blendings which must have occurred long before the Roman settlement.

We are just as ignorant of the building of Stonehenge as are the Polynesians of the erection of the trilithon of Tonga and the images of Easter Island.

Further, our own history betrays exactly the same blindness to early influences which I suppose to be present in Polynesian traditions. If we remind ourselves of the early English history we learnt at school, we shall find it almost exclusively composed of the traditions of Saxon and Norman invading kings; and indeed it is only by quite recent research that historians are coming to recognize how small a part these persons have taken in the real history of England, and how great has been the continuity with earlier institutions. Our own history gives us the clue to a feature of Folk-memory which goes far to explain the excessive weight laid by Polynesian tradition upon a feature of their history which was only the last of a series of invasions and blendings. Moreover, it is probable that the movements thus recorded in the memories of the people are not even those of the incoming of the latest of the main streams of immigration into Polynesia, but are rather records of secondary movements within the Pacific, which were perhaps the reverberations of disturbances set up in the Malay Archipelago at this time by the Hindu invasion to which are due the great temples of Java and many other signs of Hindu influence.

If the traditions of Maori or Polynesian are studied closely, it is found that they do not ignore the presence of an earlier population, though, as is customary in the traditions of conquering or predominant peoples, they tend to belittle the part played by influences other than their own. Mr Elsdon Best has recently recorded definite traditions about the indigenous peoples of New Zealand, and has shown that these traditions are in agreement with the physical diversity of the Maori people even at the present time.

It has not been possible to give all the evidence in favour

of the views I have put forward, but even if I had been able to give all the evidence, the hypothetical nature of my scheme would still have to be acknowledged. I do not claim to do more than outline a scheme which co-ordinates the known facts of Polynesian culture and will, I hope, serve to stimulate research. Does it not add interest to the study of the peoples who once held sole sway in these islands that they have preserved customs and beliefs allied to, if not derived from, one of the most wonderful civilizations which the world has ever seen ?

The researches of Mr Elsdon Best show that there are still to be found Maoris who preserve with fidelity the memories of custom and belief transmitted to them by their fathers and other instructors of their youth. His collection of records furnishes a bright gleam from the past which should encourage further efforts to recover all that yet remains in the memories of the people before it is too late. And this work should not be limited to New Zealand, but should extend to other parts of the Pacific and primarily to those places, such as the Cook Islands and Niue, the government of which has now been taken over by New Zealand. If New Zealand were to undertake a full ethnographic survey of the indigenous races over which she rules, she would make for herself a proud place in the history of science and would set an example to the other ruling peoples of the world, and not least to the mother-country, whose rulers are now only beginning faintly to recognize the responsibility which rests upon them of trying to understand the peoples over whom they have been called to rule. There is still time for New Zealand to be first in the field, to undertake the task of providing for posterity a record of customs and beliefs which are not merely of the greatest interest in themselves, but, will take no small share in building up our knowledge of the history of the human race.

X

IRRIGATION AND THE CULTIVATION OF TARO

Mr W. J. Perry has shown,[1] that the distribution of terraced cultivation and irrigation corresponds closely with that of megalithic monuments, sun-cult, mummification of the dead, and other elements of culture which seem to have been carried over the earth by one migration or connected series of migrations. He proposes the addition of a special form of agriculture to the already long list of customs and objects which Elliot Smith believes to have been distributed widespread throughout the earth.[2]

Mr Perry's conclusion rests on a rough survey of the distribution of irrigation. Here, as in the case of other elements of the megalithic complex, we need a more intensive study of the different areas of distribution in order to place the conclusion on thoroughly secure foundations. Through the kind help of the Rev. F. G. Bowie, I am now able to do this with a fair measure of completeness for the New Hebrides. Mr Bowie has sent me a number of valuable notes, based partly on personal observation in the island of Santo, partly on information given to him by the natives who come to Tongoa from most parts of the archipelago to be trained at the institution of which Mr Bowie is the head.

The first point shown by Mr Bowie's notes is the intimate connection between irrigation and the cultivation of *Colocasia esculenta*, the taro of the Polynesians. The practice of irriga-

---

[1] " The Geographical Distribution of Terraced Cultivation and Irrigation," *Mem. Proc. Manchester Lit. and Phil. Soc.*, vol. 60, 1915-16.
[2] *The Migrations of Early Culture*, Manchester, 1915.

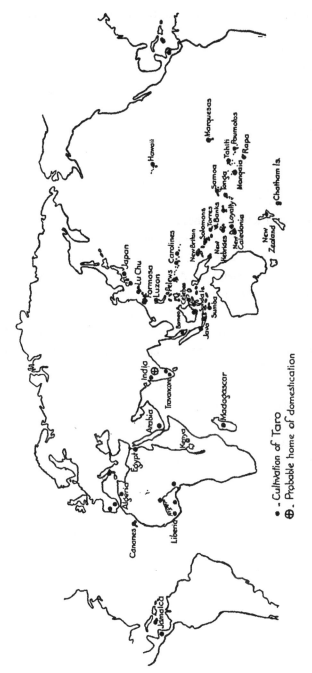

Marquesas
Hawaii
Paumotos
Tahiti
Rapa
Samoa
Tonga
Mangaia
Chatham Is.
Solomons
Torres
New Banks
New Hebrides
Loyalty
New Caledonia
New Zealand
New Britain
Japan
Lu Chu
Formosa
Luzon
Pelews Carolines
Celebes
Borneo
Sumba
Java
India
India
Travancore
Madagascar
Arabia
Kenya
Egypt
Algeria
Canaries
Liberia
Jamaica

● - Cultivation of Taro
⊕ - Probable home of domestication

CHART OF THE SITES MENTIONED BY DR RIVERS.

tion forms part, but only part, of the process of cultivation of taro.

The first part of this chapter will consist of an account of the cultivation of this food-plant in the New Hebrides. In these islands taro, which has a variety of native names, is cultivated in two ways, which may be called the wet and the dry methods. In the first method the water of springs or streams is led along channels, formed with the aid of stones, to the taro fields or beds, which are found either on relatively flat pieces of ground or on terraces artificially constructed on the sides of hills.

The construction of these channels is often assisted by artificial levelling of the ground over which they pass.

Irrigated taro fields or beds are of two kinds. In some cases, as in the island of Anaiteum, there are large level areas, in which the production of the level has probably been assisted by artificial means. In places, as in N. W. Santo, taro is cultivated on terraces which differ little in level if the slope of the ground is slight, but may be separated by several feet from one another if they have been made on a steep hill-side. The water is conducted from the channels to terrace after terrace till the whole has been irrigated. Great care is taken that the channels shall remain intact, and they are never allowed to become blocked so that the water in them becomes stagnant. The same irrigated land is used year after year, the tops of the rhizomes, dug up for food, being cut off and planted.

The dry method of cultivation resembles that used in order to grow yams except, of course, that it is not necessary to set up stakes or other objects on which to train the vines of the yam. When a piece of ground is cleared and cleaned of weeds, men dig holes with long digging sticks, and the women break up the earth with their fingers and plant the tops of the taro, which have been previously put in water for several days. In the dry method a fresh piece of ground is used every year, as in the cultivation of yams.

The distribution of the two methods of cultivating taro in the New Hebrides is largely dependent on the presence of streams or springs, but the relation between the presence of water and irrigation is not constant, for irrigation may be absent where streams are abundant. Thus, in the island of Santo, irrigation and terraced cultivation are only found to the west of a line running from north to south through the middle of the island. To the east of this line only the dry method is practised,[1] while to the west of the line both methods occur.

The absence of irrigation in the north-eastern part of the island about Hog Harbour can be explained by the absence of water, but farther southwards there is no irrigation on this side of the island, though streams are abundant. Mr Bowie says that the soil of this district seems to hold the water for a long time, and it may be that irrigation is not practised because the soil furnished sufficient moisture to allow a good crop without it. In the south of the island of Tongoa, the people irrigate : they say that the use of the dry method would only mean throwing the taro away.

In the western half of Santo both the dry and wet methods are practiced, the former especially where there are no streams, as on the hills behind Nogugu on the northern part of the coast. The dry method may also be used where there are streams, but irrigation is more usual. The area under irrigation is very large, both about Nogugu and on the western half of Big Bay. The western half of the island is very hilly with plentiful streams, and the relative sparseness of vegetation on this coast suggests that the ground is much drier than on the eastern side of the island. The character of the soil is

---

[1] Mr Bowie is uncertain about the eastern side of Big Bay (formerly called the Bay of St Philip and St James) and the valley of Ora river (usually known as the Jordan).

probably such as to make irrigation necessary if taro is to be grown with any measure of success.

In the island of Malo, at the south-eastern corner of Santo, there are no streams, water percolating into the rocky soil and reaching the lower parts of the island at swamps near the sea-shore. Owing to this absence of water and the dry character of the soil taro is hardly grown at all, and only by the dry method. Taro is the staple food of Omba (Leper's Island), but I do not know the mode of cultivation which is practised. I only know of the presence of irrigation in Maewo (Aurora) from Dr Codrington [1] who quotes Bishop Selwyn that " every inch that was available was used for irrigation, by means of one little streamlet which is made to do a vast deal of work before it can reach the sea in a course of about two miles."

On Pentecost Island, irrigation is said to be practiced in several places, but I know nothing about the details.

We do not at present know of the presence either of terraces or irrigation in Malekula, and taro seems to be of relatively little importance in this island. Mr Bowie has not heard of irrigation in the north-eastern part of the island, and Mr J. W. Layard, who worked during 1914 in the small islands off the north-eastern coast of Malekula, tells me that taro is not grown there or on the adjacent part of the coast of the main island, though the people greatly appreciate the plant as food whenever they can obtain it from the island of Omba. At present we know practically nothing about the customs of the people of the north-western part of the island, the so-called Big Nambas, and little more about the southern part of the island. It is possible that taro and irrigation may yet be found in these parts of Malekula.

In several parts of the actively volcanic island of Ambrim, taro is grown by the dry method, but the island has no streams

---

[1] See note on p. 226.

which it would be possible to use for the purpose of irrigation.

I have no information about Epi, but on Tongoa taro is not grown now. Formerly it was cultivated by the dry method, chiefly in one district of the island.

Until lately, taro was grown by the dry method on the island of Mae or Emae (Two Hills) but has been given up owing to the labour involved. There is a tradition that formerly there was a stream on the island, the water of which was utilized to irrigate taro fields.

On the island of Nguna there is no running water and only a little taro is grown by the dry method. On Fate (Sandwich Island), both methods are used.

Mr Bowie thinks that the Eromangans must practise irrigation, for two men from this island, who were formerly teachers on Santo, were great cultivators of taro. He believes also that irrigation occurs in the Kwamera district of Tanna.

On the eastern side of Futuna, in a district called Imatangi, there is a flat area, compared in size with the island of Tongoa, where taro is grown year after year by means of irrigation. Water issues from the central mountain of the island, is conducted for three or four hundred yards along a channel made with stones, and then irrigates a number of beds in the flat. The water is kept running over the beds till the taro is ripe, when it is shut off and follows along the channel till it loses itself in the ground.

In the island of Anaiteum, taro is grown by both methods. The dry method differs from that practised elsewhere in the New Hebrides in that taro is planted at any time of the year, and not only at the same time as the yam. Though the dry method is freely employed, irrigation is still more frequent. Irrigated taro fields are found all over the island, the largest being at Umetch in the south. The water with which these beds are irrigated is led from four or five springs on high ground into a main channel, from which it is carried from plot to plot by smaller channels made of volcanic stones. The channels are very ancient, and formerly supplied an area four times as large as that now used.

At another place in Anaiteum, Anelgauhat, situated inland in the southern part of the island, water is conducted along a channel made of volcanic and coral stones for about a hundred yards, while at Nawunjai a channel runs for one and a half to two miles before it reaches the terraces over which the water is distributed. It may be noted that Anaiteum possesses many varieties of taro (" perhaps a hundred " according to Mr Bowie's informant), pointing to the great antiquity of the cultivation of the plant in this region.

The connection between irrigation and the cultivation of taro which is thus so definite in the new Hebrides is also found in other parts of Melanesia. In New Caledonia [1] terraced cultivation and irrigation are extensively practiced, and seem to have reached a degree of elaboration greater than anywhere else in Melanesia. The taro is cultivated both on the hills and in the plains. The hill-sides thus culti-vated are so extensive that in one place Glaumont calculates that the taro-beds were a hundred kilometres in length, forming row after row the whole way down the sides of a semicircular hill, giving it the appearance of a Roman amphi-theatre. The whole, together with several other hills, was irrigated by water from a single stream.

On the plains, the New Caledonian often made his taro-beds in distinctive forms, the details of which are given by Glaumont. In some cases the beds thus made in the plains were fed with water which had been already used to irrigate the mountain terraces. Taro needs shade as well as moisture, and this is obtained, both on hill and plain, by planting sugar-cane and bananas in the spaces separating the taro-beds from one another.

[1] Glaumont, L'Anthropologie, viii (1897), 46.

In the Loyalty Islands there is no water which can be used for irrigation, and little if any taro is grown.[1]

In the Banks Islands, north of the New Hebrides, taro is grown in irrigated gardens on the island of Vanua Lava. The steep sides of the conical island of Merlav have been formed into terraces on which gardens are made, but I do not know whether irrigation is practised.

In the Torres Islands, taro (*kweta*) is little used, but the fact that it gives its name to one of the months[2] suggests that it was formerly more important in the lives of the people.

The point brought out most clearly by the evidence from the New Hebrides and New Caledonia is, as I have already said, the intimate relation between irrigation and the cultivation of taro. Where irrigation is practised in these islands, it is used for the cultivation of taro, and for no other purpose.

This appears also to hold good for other parts of Melanesia and of Polynesia. The extensive irrigation of the island of Nduke or Kulambangara in the Solomons, and of certain islands of the Fijian Archipelago,[3] is used exclusively for taro ; and this also holds good of the Marquesa Islands in Polynesia.[4]

If irrigation and terraced cultivation belong to the megalithic complex, the intimate connection between these practices and the growth of taro makes it difficult to resist the conclusion that taro also belongs to this complex, and that the cultivation of this food-plant was introduced by the people who carried mummification of the dead and the other customs which have a similar distribution.

If now we inquire into the distribution of taro, we find that this plant, so closely associated in the minds of ethnologists with Oceania, really has a very wide distribution, and is used as a food in many parts of the world. According to

[1] See p. 283.
[2] I am indebted for this fact to the Rev. W. J. Durrard.
[3] A. M. Hocart, quoted by Perry, *op. cit.*, pp. 16-17.
[4] Tautain, *L'Anthropologie*, viii (1897), 542.

Reinhardt,[1] *Colocasia antiquorum* or *esculenta* is used as a food in India and eastern Asia as far north as Japan, in the Malay archipelago, in Arabia and Egypt, in East and West Africa, in Algeria, Spain and the Canary Islands, and in the tropical parts of America. According to de Candolle,[2] it is cultivated in Portugal, and also in southern Italy, where it is called " aro di Egitto."

It will be noted by all who have followed the work of Elliot Smith how closely this distribution agrees with that of the group of customs he assigns to the megalithic complex. Such attempts as I have made to study the distribution of taro more closely have not been very successful, and one of the objects of this paper is the hope that it may stimulate workers in economic botany to record more fully than they have hitherto done, not merely the presence of this food-plant, but also its mode of cultivation.

Reinhardt states that in one part of West Africa where the plant is called *dinde*, it is a staple article of food. I have not been able to identify the locality where taro is so named, but Mr N. W. Thomas tells me that under the customary name of *koko* yam, *Colocasia esculenta* is cultivated by the Ibo, Edo, Fanti and other peoples of West Africa, but he does not know of it as a staple food anywhere. It is not cultivated by means of irrigation, but is grown in swamps by women, who both plant the gardens and own the produce. The term by which *Colocasia* is widely, if not universally known in West Africa is *koko*. This word is also used in Jamaica and as M. Delafosse has pointed out to me, this suggests that the plant has reached Africa from the West Indies in recent times. It is possible, however, that the movement may have been in the other direction. In Uganda, the Rev. J. Roscoe tells me that the rhizome of an arum called *timpa* by the natives,

---

[1] *Kulturgeschichte der Nutzpflanzen*, München, 1911, p. 368.
[2] *Origin of Cultivated Plants*, London, 1884, p. 73.

which is almost certainly *Colocasia esculenta*, is grown, but it is not an important article of food. It is cultivated only by the more advanced gardeners. The plant thrives in low-lying moist land, where there is a rich loam washed down from the hills, and the ground is neither irrigated or watered. As in New Caledonia, the plant is grown in the shade of plantains.

In India, *Colocasia esculenta* is widely cultivated, being an especially common food in Travancore. I have not been able to discover how far irrigation is used in its cultivation.

In Japan taro has been cultivated since prehistoric times, both irrigation and the dry method being used.

So far, I have been able to learn very little about the cultivation of taro in America. It is an important article of food in the West Indies, but I do not know whether it is cultivated by means of irrigation. Taro is certainly a food-plant in Central and in the tropical parts of South America, but here again I know at present nothing about its mode of cultivation.

We need more knowledge of the exact details of distribution and mode of cultivation of *Colocasia esculenta* before the association of this plant with the megalithic people can be fully established, but such knowledge as we already possess points definitely towards the migrations of this people as the means by which the plant was distributed so widely over the earth. It may be noted in passing that, in this case, the evidence concerning distribution has been collected by botanists and not by ethnologists. It is a frequent reproach against the conclusions of Elliot Smith that they depend on partial surveys, and that his diagrams of distribution might have a very different appearance if we knew all the facts. The survey of distribution of *Colocasia esculenta* on which I have relied has been collected by workers quite free from any ethnological bias, and is probably as complete as that of any other plant. There is no reason to suppose that further knowledge will alter the general character of the distribution. The facts we need are rather those which do not especially interest the botanist, facts about the mode of cultivation, and its place in the religious and social life of the people, as well as more exact details concerning its importance in different districts of the regions where it is found.

One conclusion of great interest suggested by the facts given in this paper is that taro would seem to afford an example of an element of culture acquired by the megalithic people in the course of their travels and transported by them to their original home.   When it was believed, as I suppose most of us once believed, that the early migrations of man were due to lack of food, or to enemies driving him from his home, the dispersal of culture seemed a relatively simple process.   If early migrations simply spread outwards from a centre as the result of some *vis a tergo*, the stream of movement would be in one direction only.

It is one of the many important consequences of the contribution to our knowledge made by Mr Perry, in his paper on " The Relationship between the Geographical Distribution of Megalithic Monuments and Ancient Mines," [1] that this simplicity can no longer be expected.   If the impetus to the early migrations of mankind was the prospect of gaining material wealth, it follows that these migrations were of a highly complex kind, involving intercourse between distant places lasting for long periods of time, with constant movements to and fro.   In this case the movement of culture would not be a single centrifugal diffusion, but an intricate process in which elements of culture would be transported in various directions, the travellers taking to their homes, objects and customs with which they had become acquainted in the course of their travels.

So far as I am aware, we have had until now no element

[1] *Mem. and Proc. Manchester Lit. and Phil. Soc.*, vol. 60, pt. i, 1915.

of the culture of the Eastern Mediterranean which we could regard at all definitely as having been brought there from the east by the megalithic people. But if *Colocasia esculenta* belongs to the megalithic complex, there is little doubt that it is such an object. Botanists are agreed that the original home of the plant is Southern Asia, probably India, and the great variety of native names for the plant [1] in India shows that its importance in this country goes back to a remote date. If India is the original home of taro, the knowledge of its economic utility would have been acquired there by the megalithic people, and, together with the plant itself, taken thence to Egypt, Arabia and the Eastern Mediterranean. According to Reinhardt, its further dispersal westwards took place in the Middle Ages through the wanderings of the Arabs, and the fact that the South Italian name of the plant so clearly points to its source in Egypt may perhaps be regarded as evidence in favour of this late date for its movement westwards. Its presence in Algeria and the Canary Islands, and possibly also in West Africa, however, is more probably due to a far earlier migration in which taro accompanied the other manifestations of megalithic activity of which these places are the seat. It may be noted that, according to Reinhardt, *Colocasia esculenta* was known in Egypt as early as 500 B.C.

Another problem of great interest is illustrated by the facts brought forward in this place. If a culture is carried from one place to another by means of migration, an exact agreement in the distribution of its elements is most unlikely. We must expect that, for one reason or another, one element of culture will fail to take root here and another there. Other elements, again, will flourish for a time in the new home, and will then degenerate or disappear, owing to some character

---

[1] See Watt, *Dictionary of the Economic Products of India*, Calcutta, 1889, vol. ii.

S

of the new environment unsuited to their success, while still other elements will suffer such modification that it may become difficult to recognize the relation of the final product to the custom from which it is derived. Among the factors which take part in this process of differentiation, none are more important than those we may class together as geographical : conditions of climate, configuration of country, nature of soil, etc. Such elements as cultivated plants and modes of agriculture are especially likely to show the influence of these geographical factors, and the influence of some of them upon the distribution of taro is evident. Thus, taro is a plant suited to tropical and semi-tropical climates, and we cannot expect to find its distribution agreeing with that of other objects and customs carried by migrations which have extended to temperate regions.

Some of the facts brought forward in this paper bring out very clearly another factor which has greatly influenced the distribution of taro and irrigation. In the New Hebrides, it is clear that the presence of irrigation is definitely associated with certain natural conditions, with a relatively dry soil and the presence of streams. Where the soil is moist, taro is grown, but irrigation is not necessary. The absence of irrigation in certain parts of this region is clearly due either to the absence of streams or to the nature of the soil making unnecessary the arduous operations of terraced cultivation and irrigation.

A similar condition exists in Fiji. Mr Hocart tells me that on the windward side of Viti Levu, where moisture is abundant and the soil suitable for the growth of taro, irrigation does not occur, while in the eastern islands of the Fijian Archipelago, the soil is dry and irrigation is practised. Again, in Polynesia, the island of Rotuma has no streams and its people use the dry method of cultivating taro, while in the Tongan Islands, which are flat and ill-watered, irrigation is also absent.

It may be noted that in both East and West Africa where taro is grown without irrigation, the soil is moist and adapted to the dry method.

My task thus far has been to show that if irrigation and terraced cultivation belong to the group of customs distributed by the migrations which carried the megalithic art and mummification of the dead, the use of taro must also be included in the group. This conclusion, based originally upon the close connection of irrigation with the cultivation of taro in Oceania, has received striking confirmation from a study of the distribution of the plant. This distribution has hitherto, I believe, been wholly unnoticed by the ethnologist, but its general agreement with that of so many other elements of culture greatly adds to the strength of the position held by Elliot Smith and Perry.

I propose now to leave the topic of the general distribution of irrigation and the cultivation of taro, and consider in more detail the evidence from Southern Melanesia. The conclusions of Elliot Smith and Perry are based on a general survey of the distribution of certain objects and customs over the earth. In order fully to establish their position, it will be necessary to subject each of the areas of this distribution to an intensive study in order to ascertain how far the details of distribution can be brought into harmony with the conclusions suggested by the more general survey.

The New Hebrides and New Caledonia show definite signs of the presence of the megalithic culture, dolmen-like structures of stones taking an important place in their ceremonial. In the New Hebrides, two places are especially characterized by the extent and elaborateness of irrigation, the north-eastern part of Santo and the island of Anaiteum, and in the former locality the dolmen-like structures to which I have referred are especially definite. I have not visited Anaiteum, the other chief centre of irrigation, but this island is the seat of representations of the sun and moon in stone which suggest the strong influence of the megalithic culture.

On the other hand, irrigation is, so far as we know, absent in the island of Malekula, where the dolmen-like structures and other manifestations of megalithic activity are more definite and elaborate than in any other part of the archipelago. As the evidence stands at present, the common distribution of irrigation and megalithic elements holds good to a certain extent in the New Hebrides, but breaks down at a most important point.

While the evidence from the New Hebrides is thus inconclusive, New Caledonia affords a striking example of the association of irrigation and terraced cultivation with the megalithic culture. The irrigation of this island surpasses in extent and elaboration anything recorded from other parts of Melanesia, and this island has also preserved more completely than any other part of this area the complex of customs assigned by Elliot Smith and Perry to the megalithic culture, possessing as it does no less than nine of these elements, namely, stone monuments, mummification, sun-cult, sacred chieftainship, incision, tattooing, distension of the ear-lobes, deformation of the head and irrigation. The association of the most complete irrigation known in Melanesia with the most complete preservation of the megalithic complex found in this area, affords striking evidence in favour of the view of Elliot Smith and Perry.

While the distribution of irrigation and of the more extensive cultivation of taro thus shows a general agreement with that of the megalithic culture in the New Hebrides and New Caledonia, the island of Malekula forms an exception for which we must account before the main position can be fully established. It is already possible to see the lines by which this obstacle can be removed, but as they are derived from evidence collected by Mr Layard and myself which has not yet been published it will only be possible here to give the general outlines of the argument by which this problem may be solved. The distribution of funeral customs in Polynesia points to the presence of two megalithic immigrations into this area, an earlier which brought the practice of mummification of the dead on platforms and a later which practised interment in the extended position in vaults. The earlier influence is especially apparent in the more eastern and northern islands of Polynesia, such as the Marquesas, Tahiti and the Hawaiian Islands, while the later is most evident in the Tongan and Samoan groups in the west.

When dealing with Melanesia in my book,[1] I discerned a similar double influence, especially in the Banks and Torres Islands, but the evidence then at my disposal was insufficient to allow me to speak positively on this point, or to assign other elements of culture to the two influences. A visit to the New Hebrides since my book was written has shown conclusively that this archipelago has been the seat of a process whereby the preservation of the dead by rude kinds of mummification has gone altogether into the background in favour of interment of the dead in the extended position, often with the use of stone in such a manner as to suggest the survivals of the use of a vault or of some idea connected with stone of which the vault of Samoa and Tonga was one manifestation. Moreover, it is now possible to connect these two modes of disposal of the dead with different kinds of stone monument and with different groups of objects and customs, though only when the facts collected by Mr Layard and myself have been studied more fully will it be possible to carry out the process of analysis completely.

I have now to consider how far this distinction of two strata of the megalithic culture in Southern Melanesia is capable of solving the difficulty provided by the absence of irrigation in Malekula. In the northern part of this island

---

[1] *History of Melanesian Society*, 2 Vols Cambridge, 1914.

and in the numerous small islands which fringe its north-eastern coast, we have the clearest indications of the influence which I suppose to have introduced the practice of interment in the extended position, while in the southern part of Male-kula, in Santo, Anaiteum and New Caledonia, this influence is either absent or far less evident. The absence of irrigation in the island which shows the greatest influence of the later migration and its high degree of development in islands where this later influence is absent or of small extent, points to the association of irrigation and the cultivation of taro with the earlier of the two migrations. The absence of irrigation in Malekula and the small importance of taro must be explained either by the earlier migration having had little influence in this island or to the earlier culture having been displaced by the later influence. In the latter case we should expect to find in Malekula traces of an ancient system of irrigation, but this island has been so little explored that it is not at present possible to say whether such traces do or do not exist. There is evidence from many parts of the New Hebrides that irrigation and the cultivation of taro have become far less important than in former times, and there is reason to suppose that the disuse of taro is to be connected with an increasing use of the yam, which does not require an especially moist soil or any laborious system of irrigation.

The evidence from southern Melanesia pointing to the connection of irrigation and the cultivation of taro with the earlier of the two megalithic invasions is supported by the conditions existing in Polynesia. The cultivation of taro on irrigated terraces is especially characteristic of the more eastern islands where the bodies of dead chiefs are preserved on platforms, and the associated customs of irrigation and mummification are especially developed in the Marquesas, the most eastern and outlying of the larger island-groups of Polynesia. In the Samoan and Tongan Islands, on the other hand, where the bodies of chiefs are interred in vaults in the extended position after a period of exposure which may be a survival of preservation on platforms, the cultivation of taro is either absent as in Tonga or is not grown by means of irrigation, and is less important than other kinds of food.

It is a striking fact that, both in Polynesia and Southern Melanesia, irrigation and the cultivation of taro should have flourished especially in outlying islands such as the Marquesas, the Paumotus New Caledonia, Anaiteum and Santo.

The distribution in Polynesia suggests an older culture characterized by the practices of preserving the dead on platforms, and cultivating taro by terraced irrigation, into which there has intruded from the west a people who interred their dead in the extended position, and substituted other foods and modes of agriculture for the growth of taro by irrigation. The distribution of these elements of culture in Melanesia, on the other hand, suggests that the later intrusion occurred chiefly in the central island of Malekula, and did not reach, or had much less influence, in the outlying islands of Santo, Anaiteum and New Caledonia.

I have assumed throughout this inquiry that the similarities of culture found in different parts of the earth have been produced by transmission from one place to another. I may conclude by considering briefly how far the facts I have brought forward are capable of explanation on the alternative hypothesis of independent origin.

I have shown that the presence of taro and its mode of cultivation are dependent in several parts of Oceania upon geographical conditions, and this dependence might well be regarded as evidence in favour of independent origin. According to this hypothesis, the general distribution of *Colocasia esculenta* would depend on factors similar to those which have determined the distribution of other plants, and whether it has or has not been cultivated in any one region would depend on the suitability of the geographical environment for its cultivation. According to the hypothesis, the people of different parts of the world were led or driven to the discovery of irrigation and terraced cultivation whenever the character of the soil was unsuited to the simpler modes of cultivation. Here, as in the case of the rival hypothesis, it will not do to be content with vague generalizations. The distribution of customs must be studied intensively to see how far the details accord with the hypothesis.

We have seen that the distribution of the cultivation of taro by irrigation in Southern Melanesia provided a difficulty for the hypothesis of transmission in company with the megalithic culture, a difficulty which I have sought to remove by means of a subsidiary hypothesis. This subsidiary hypothesis not only goes far towards solving the Melanesian problem, but explains even more satisfactorily the similar conditions presented by the distribution of taro, and its cultivation by irrigation in Polynesia. I have now to inquire how far the difficulty raised by the absence of irrigation in Malekula can be explained on the hypothesis of its independent origin in Southern Melanesia.

From all we know of Malekula it would seem to be well-suited to the cultivation of taro by irrigation. The absence of irrigation cannot be explained by difference of climate, for the practice is found both to the north and south, nor can it be explained by difference of altitude or watering, for in both respects Malekula closely resembles Santo, where the cultivation of taro by irrigation is so extensively practised. If we turn from climate and configuration of country to the people, we are in no better case, for the inhabitants of Malekula differ little in physical character from those Melanesians who grow taro by irrigation, and there is no reason whatever to suppose that there are such mental differences as would be necessary to explain the failure to react to conditions so similar to those which, according to the hypothesis, have produced the practices of irrigation and terraced cultivation in other islands. The general social culture of Malekula differs from that of other islands of Melanesia in certain respects which I have already considered. The advocates of independent origin ought to be able to tell us why those peoples of Southern Melanesia who preserved their dead on platforms and discovered certain rude forms of mummification, should also have discovered and elaborated to so high a degree the arts of irrigation and terraced cultivation. They ought also to be able to tell us why other peoples of so similar physical and mental character should have been led to inter their dead in the extended position at or about the same time as it was found that the yam provided a more profitable and less troublesome crop than taro. Only when the advocates of independent origin have dealt with such topics as these and have shown why such apparently disconnected processes as the growth of taro by irrigation and mummification of the dead should be associated, will their guiding .idea become more than a vague and empty speculation.

TARO IN POLYNESIA [1]

Marquesas. Mentioned by TAUTAIN (*L'Anthropologie*, VIII, 1897, 542, 548).
> Also by E. S. C. HANDY (*The Native Culture in the Marquesas*, Honolulu, 1923, 182). Terraced irrigation employed.

Tahiti. W. ELLIS, *Polynesian Researches*, 1829, I, 357. No mention of irrigation.

Laivaivai. MOERENHOUT, I, 140.

Rapa. MOERENHOUT, I, 135, 381.

Mangaia. GILL, *Jottings*, 197.

Hawaii. DAVID MALO, *Hawaiian Antiquities*, Honolulu, 1903.

Samoa. STAIR, *Old Samoa*, 1897. Grown. No mention of irrigation, 58, 129, 147.
> TURNER, *Samoa*, 42, 43, 105.
> LESSON, *Poly.*, II, 476 seq.

---

[1] Based on Rivers's notes.

Tonga. MARINER, 1817, II, 285-6.

New Zealand. T. F. CHEESEMAN, *T.N.Z.I.*, XXXIII
(1901), 306. Taro is believed to have been brought to
New Zealand by the Maori, together with the sweet
potato, the gourd and the paper mulberry. Fifty years
ago it was seen in almost every Maori cultivation of any
size, but has now fallen into almost total disuse.
   Mr Elsdon Best, in reply to an inquiry from Rivers,
made the following statement:—" There are few traditions about the taro. The ritual, myths, etc. noted in
Maori agricultural operations clustered round the Kumara,
the mythical origin of which is assigned to one Pani, a
female being, who gave birth to the Kumara in water
always, a curious occurrence, it being grown on dry land
areas.   Have old myths connected with a food plant
grown in water or wet ground been transferred to a dry
land product ?   The taro was here grown on ordinary
alluvial flats as well as damp places, such as near streams.
I saw it still growing *in* streams in the far north near old
long-deserted native cultivations.   But very little taro is
now grown, the potato has taken its place, also that of
the Kumara.   It was never grown on irrigated land by
the Maori of New Zealand.   I have 36 names of varieties
(Maori) but several names doubtless were applied to each
variety—in different districts. Taro was planted in
shallow round holes and gravel was carried from pit or
riverside and spread round plants."
   SKINNER in *The Material Culture of the Moriori of the
Chatham Islands*, states that taro was introduced by the
first immigrants, but that it is remembered now only in
tradition.

MELANESIA

Fiji. The following are extracts from a letter from Hocart
   to Rivers (16th May 1916) :—
   " In Fiji they have the Tailevu or dry land method ;
the taro is planted on the hill-side, often intermixed with
yams. The ' islands ' method is irrigation. Whatever
may be the origin of the two they have little or no ethnological significance now ; they are imposed by conditions.
On the windward side of Viti Levu, alias Tailevu, the
moisture is abundant and the soil suitable.   The islands
lack moisture and the soil is often hard.   Taro is rare on
the Leeward side of Viti Levu, but I have unfortunately
not noted the method used there.
   " I have seen terraces in Ovalau, and Tavenui. In
Lakemoa there are none, the reason evidently being that

there is hardly any sloping taro land. Rotuma, which
has no water, uses the dry land method ; Wallis, which is
flat, irrigates, if I remember well. . . . Irrigation is said
to have been a frequent cause of quarrels in old Lakemba."

Malekula (New Hebrides). The following is an extract from
a letter written by Mr E. G. McAfee of South-West
Bay, Malekula, to Mr John Layard, who worked in the
neighbourhood with Rivers in 1914 :—" So far as I
can find out, taro is not planted in terraces, but irrigation is used in a few places. I know of only two, Belias
and Lotaha (Meaun district). At these places the whole
village uses the irrigation works in common. In other
places a native makes a taro garden wherever he finds
suitable wet land. There are several kinds of taro, and
they are planted according to the amount of moisture in
the land, the taro growing in land flooded with water
being the largest and best. The bushmen grow more
taro than the shore natives. It seems that the interior
of the island is more suitable for taro gardens. . . . At
Seniang (where you spent most of your time) little or no
taro is grown, but further east of there, where the hills
are lower, a little is grown. I know of one place where
it is grown in red clay."

Loyalty Islands. Rivers (p. 269) states that little, if any, taro is
grown in the Loyalty Islands. But Mr E. Hadfield records
the practice :—" The large swamp of Urea offers a
splendid field for this tuber. The Lipuans also grow it." [1]

Solomon Islands. " In Guadalcanar very little is grown on the
coast, but the bush folk are taro growers " (letter from
Mr Rudolph Sprott to Rivers). " Taro is the chief
article of food on Ysabel, and the people there would, I
think, cultivate it better than any others ; for I think
that on the whole they are a higher type than the rest of
the Solomons people " (idem).

Writing from Bogotu in Ysabel, Mr Edmond Bourne
says that taro " is certainly the staple food of Ysabel,
particularly of the bush villages, among the mountains."
He goes on to say that he knows of no terracing in the
island :—" I should imagine that the special conditions to
account for the absence of terracing in Ysabel would
probably be (speaking without the book) that in our
mountains the rainfall is heavier, and mountain rivulets
more numerous, so that natural irrigation supersedes
the artificial, and also the soil of parts at least of Ysabel
may be better suited to the cultivation of taro." [2]

[1] E. Hadfield, *Among the Natives of the Loyalty Group*, London, 1920.
[2] See also Codrington, *The Melanesians*, 304, 319.

Taro is cultivated in New Britain, and irrigation is practised where practicable.[1]

CAROLINE ISLANDS

Taro is cultivated in the Caroline Islands[2] and in the Pelews.[3] It is mentioned further north in the Lu Chu group.[4]

THE PHILIPPINES

The Bontoc Igorot cultivate taro, but rarely. It is more common outside their area. Taro is closely associated with Lumawig, their culture-hero, who came from the sky. He first taught the Bontoc agriculture, and in his garden some taro is kept growing.[5]

INDONESIA

There is a certain amount of information concerning the growing of *taro* in Indonesia. Wilken, in his *Handleiding voor de Vergelijkende Volkenkunds van Nederlandsch-Indie*[6] mentions it among the Malays, also in Java, the Sunda Islands and among the Olo Ngadju of south-east Borneo. (See Hardeland Dajacksch-Deutsches Worterbuch, s.v. *kudjang*). But the most definite information comes from Kruyt. He states that *Colocasia* is cultivated in the whole of central and north Celebes, including Minahassa. It is generally planted near to houses, and not, as in the case of other plants, in the rice-fields. A wild kind is found, but is not eaten.[7] The Bare'e Toradja use taro when the rice fails.[8] An old man among the To Ondae, the oldest Toradja people, told how in very old times at Wawo Tolo, one of their first villages, a funeral feast was given at which taro alone was eaten. "All that we can conclude from this tale is that *Colocasia* was formerly grown in larger quantities and was more prized." At present guests are only given *Colocasia* when the rice-crops have failed.[9]

The people of the Mountain Toradja used taro. "They

---

[1] E. Brown, *Melanesians and Polynesians*, 125, 325.
[2] F. W. Christian, *The Caroline Islands*, pp. 338, 342, 347, 350, 351.
[3] J. Kubary, *Ethnographische Beitrage zur Kentniss des Karolinen Archipelo*, Leiden, 1895, 156; see G. Keate, *Account of Pelew Islands and Journals, etc., of Capt. Henry Wilson*, 1788, p. 299.
[4] Julien de la Gravière, *Voyage en Chine*, i, 232.
[5] A. E. Jenks, *The Bontoc Igorot*, 139, 140, 202.
[6] Leiden, 1893.
[7] Letter from Kruyt to Perry.
[8] A. C. Kruyt, *De Bare'e aprekende Toradjas van Midden-Celebes*, 's-Gragenhage, 1912, ii, 203.
[9] Letter to Perry.

told me in Napu, and each inhabitant that I asked confirmed it, that they formerly used *Colocasia* before they knew of rice. *Colocasia* is there also an important part of the offerings made to the gods. A tale collected by Kruyt suggests that formerly taro was cooked in ovens as in Polynesia. The To Napu use taro in time of scarcity. Kruyt also states that only the nobility eat rice, and that the commoners have to eat taro and yams.[1]

Sumba. Kruyt mentions also that taro is grown in Sumba.[2]

Formosa. In Formosa the natives plant taro on their terraces. They prefer irrigated terraces. The planting time is in February, and the crop is gathered in June and July. In Japan taro has been cultivated from prehistoric times, both by irrigation and the dry methods. The cultivation is especially well developed in the Southern and Eastern parts.[3]

INDIA

The following is an extract from information sent by Mr F. J. Richards:—" Regarding its distribution it may be said that it is found all over this Presidency (Madras), and in Bombay to a great extent. . . . Both in Bombay and Madras Presidencies this is grown as a field crop in garden lands under well or canal irrigation. . . . In Madras and Bombay Presidencies this is favoured by all castes of people as a vegetable."

MADAGASCAR

W. D. MAROUSE. *Through Western Madagascar.* London, 1914, p. 317, mentions *Colocasia esculenta* as grown in every native compound. The same writer in a letter written to Rivers (25th Jan. 1917), mentions that it is grown " on the mud residue of the flood waters of the Madagascar Rivers. There is no irrigation in a European sense, only a crude native " lift by bamboo."

AFRICA

East Africa Protectorate. A letter from Mr C. W. Hobley writes:—" *Colocasia esculenta* is very largely grown in this country, but not at low altitudes. It flourishes in Kikuyu particularly, and also in the higher parts of Kavirondo. I think I have seen it in the Taita Hill, and

---

[1] Letter to Perry: *op. cit.*, ii, 203.
[2] A. C. Kruyt, " Verslag van eene reis over het eiland Soemba," *Tijdschrift van het Kon. Nederlandsch Aardrijkskundig Genootschap*, 2nd ser., pt. xxxviii, 1921, 535.
[3] Information of Mr Shinji Ishii to Perry.

I believe it grows in Chagga. It is usually grown in the river valleys, in the small strip of alluvium on each side of the streams in Kikuyu. . . . Irrigation is used to a small extent in Taita and Kikuyu and to a considerable extent in Chagga, but not specially in connection with the growth of *Colocasia*. The natives do not plant fields of it, but one will find a dozen roots here and there where the soil is suitable." [1]

SCHWEINFURTH, *Heart of Africa*, I, p. 211, mentions *Colocasia* as cultivated freely throughout the Niam-Niam country. See also p. 282.

West Africa. In West Africa *Colocasia esculenta* is widely grown.

Southern Nigeria. (PARTRIDGE, *Cross River Natives*, 1905, p. 149). In a letter, Mr N. W. Thomas writes that *Colocasia esculenta* " is a common food in most places— Edo, Ibo, Fanti, etc., but nowhere, so far as I know, a staple. It is usually cultivated by women. . . . If a man fails to grow enough yams in the Edo country, he will live on koko yams (*Colocasia esculenta.*) " M. Delafosse writes to Rivers from Dakar:—" I have met *Colocasia* cultivated in nearly every part of the Ivory Coast Colony and also along the Black Volta, in the French and British territories of High Senegal-Niger and the Gold Coast. But my very, very small knowledge in botanical matters does not make me able to ascertain if the plant I have seen, without appreciable solution of continuity, from the sea as far as the eleventh parallel, is everywhere of the same variety. The only one thing I can say is that it appeared to me as the same one and cultivated in the same way. As for its frequency, I have noticed it to be in larger quantity between the parallels 5th and 7th (forest region), only sporadic between the 7th and 9th and more frequent between the 9th and 11th parallels. Nowhere is it the basis of native food, except perhaps on the borders of the low Tanoe, along the boundary-line between the Ivory and Gold Coasts, where yams are scarce and food especially consists of plantains and ' coco ' (*Colocasia esculenta*). It is worthy of remark that in nearly all the coast languages that plant—or rather its eatable part—is named ' coco,' which is the name given to it in the West Indies. That would seem to be an indication that *Colocasia esculenta* has been imported from America. I heard the word ' coco ' is also used to design it in Yucatan. I met the same plant

[1] H. H. Johnston, *Tu Kihma-Njan Expedition*, i, 1886, 124, 139, 149, 441, 442.

largely cultivated in Liberia, all along the coast, under the same name of ' coco ' as well by the natives as by the Liberians. In French Sudan and, in the Niger Valley, the plant is met with here and there and cultivated by natives who, I must say, do not appreciate it very much. I never noticed any way of irrigation or special cultivation used. It is only said the plant needs a wet soil and does not give good produce in dry country."

PART IV

GENERAL

I

TRADE, WARFARE, AND SLAVERY

I PROPOSE to consider some examples of social activity which are generally included under the headings of trade, warfare and slavery, with the object of showing how greatly these concepts, when applied to comparatively simple societies, may differ in their nature from what we are accustomed to in our own society. In all three examples, we shall find the common feature that social processes which among ourselves may have functions almost exclusively economic or political, may in other societies be as intimately linked with religious or magical significations.

I will begin with trade and will take as my chief example the institution of the south-eastern archipelago of New Guinea called *Kula*.[1]

Some of the islands of this archipelago are fertile and grow extensive crops, while others are rocky islets on which food sufficient for the needs of the inhabitants cannot be grown. These smaller islands are the seat of definite industries, such as the making of pottery and canoe-building, while the commodities so produced are bartered for the food of the larger and more fertile islands. At first sight, it would appear that we have a simple example of trade carried on with a definite and obvious motive, and yet Malinowski has shown that this process of barter is merely the accompaniment of a highly ceremonial process of exchanging articles which have no intrinsic value. The exchange of these useless articles

[1] See B. Malinowski, *The Argonauts of the Western Pacific*, 1922.

is a highly complex affair and follows certain rules of a ceremonial kind.   There is reason to believe that if this ceremonial exchange fell into disorder, the more useful process of
barter which acts as a subsidiary feature of the ceremonial
exchange would be seriously impaired or even destroyed.

The articles which are thus ceremonially exchanged are
only two in number, arm-shells and necklaces composed of
strings of shell-discs.   Each article passes from one community
to another, according to definite rules.   The arm-shells must
always travel to the south from the place Malinowski takes
as his starting-point, while the shell-discs travel to the north.
Moreover, these two articles are always on the move and
never stay for any length of time with one owner, but must
be passed on at the danger of serious reproach for what we
can only call a breach of honour or commercial integrity.
The whole transaction is intimately connected with the idea
that liberality is one of the highest of virtues while meanness
brings shame and social opprobrium upon the miser.   Considerable complication is introduced into the whole business
by the fact that the exchange does not occur as one transaction, but if I visit another place taking with me an armlet,
I do not at once receive in exchange the necklet of shell-
discs.   This may only be received, perhaps a year later, when
the man who received my armlet pays me a visit, and as it
is definitely recognized that all armlets and necklaces are not
equal in value, there is the further complication that intermediate gifts may be necessary while awaiting the full
exchange, or that subsidiary offerings may be made if a person
desires to obtain an armlet or necklace of especial fineness.
Certain of the objects which thus circulate are so fine that
they have special individual names and are known to all, so
that a definite impression is produced in a district when one
of these well-known objects reaches it.

So far as we know, this institution of the *kula*, described

by Malinowski, is unique, but there are many features of
Melanesian trade which fit in with the general conception.
Throughout Melanesia, exchange of a more or less ceremonial
kind forms a prominent feature of every religious rite, while
a complicated system of what can only be regarded as
exchange forms an equally prominent feature of the ritual of
the graded organizations usually known as secret societies.
There is clear evidence that the objects used in this exchange
are usually called money, and I may take this opportunity of
saying a few words about the institution of money. Dr
Malinowski has rejected the view that the objects which
circulate during the *kula* are to be regarded as money, and
quite rightly, for they have none of its distinguishing features.
The so-called money of Melanesia is of two chief kinds. In
the Solomons, the chief currency takes the forms of arm-rings
of shell, apparently similar to those of the *Kula* of the
Trobriands, but they are definitely used as intermediums in
transactions in which some other object passes from one
person to another. A certain number will be given in exchange
for a pig, for instance, and they are used in the transactions
accompanying marriage. They can definitely be regarded as
currency, acting as an object through the intermediation of
which exchange is effected. Moreover, the rings are graded
in value, and three chief kinds are recognized, the most
valuable being a large arm-ring called *mbakia*, made from the
shell of the giant clam, which has a special yellow mark.
The next is a ring called *poata* of the same kind without such
a mark, while the third is a section of a trochus shell called
mbokalo, which is both smaller in size and slighter in form.
Moreover, there is a definite scale of values ; a *mbakia* is worth
two *poata*, and a *poata* is worth ten *mbokalo*. In fact, the
young Solomon islander could be given a table of money to
learn, exactly comparable with our own.

In the Banks Islands, the objects used in the graded

organizations correspond even more closely with the definition of money. They consist of strings of small shell-discs. Those of a red colour have a greater value than those that are white, but a more definite means by which payments are graduated is through the length of the piece of string of shell-discs which passes from one person to another. The chief unit is the fathom, but other smaller units are used, including that called *chiregi*, which is measured from one shoulder to the tip of the fingers of the other arm, amounting to about four feet. Another is the cubit, measured from the elbow to the tip of the outstretched fingers, while a still shorter unit is from the wrist to the end of the fingers.

In this concise graduation and use of definite units of value, the shell-discs can definitely be regarded as money, but they are certainly more prominent as part of the complicated exchanges of the graded organizations than in buying food. It seems also that exchange of this kind by means of which the money passes from the islands where it is made into general circulation is far more frequent than its use as an intermediary object in obtaining food within the society formed by the inhabitants of an island or village.

A more difficult case is provided by the mats and pigs, which are the only objects which can possibly be regarded as money in the New Hebrides. Here the mats certainly are only used in ceremonial transactions, and this is also largely true of the pigs. Every ceremony, including that of initiation into a graded organization or into a higher rank of these organizations, involves not also the passage of pigs from one person to another, but, since there is a definite scale of values, chiefly dependent on the length of the tusk, they may also be regarded as money, though of a less definite kind perhaps than the armlets of the Solomons or the shell-discs of the Banks Islands.

The chief use of these forms of money, and especially of

the money of the Banks Islands and New Hebrides is without any doubt ceremonial, and it is significant that the term for the money of Melanesia often means "sacred," examples of this being the *rongo* of the Solomon Islands and the *tambu* of New Britain and Duke of York Island. It is clear that in Melanesia generally, as in the Trobriands, the primary meaning of the objects we class with our money is religious or magical, while its more strictly economic use is a subsidiary function.

There is plenty of evidence that a ceremonial exchange of goods occurs in North America and is especially characteristic of the potlatch of the North-Western tribes, while it is a question whether there may not be ideas or sentiments of somewhat the same kind as those of Melanesia behind the numerous transactions with cattle in Africa.

There is reason to believe that when a native is growing his crops, what is most prominent in his mind is not their use as food, but their value in ceremony and as a means of showing the liberality which is so prominent in his conception of social behaviour.

Trade provides an example of social processes taking place between the members of different societies and I shall take as my next example another process, of a very different kind, which takes place between rather than within societies.

There is little doubt, again, that the warfare of comparatively simple societies is often largely ceremonious. I will take the warfare of Eddystone Island in the Solomons as an instance. Here, there are two different kinds of warfare— one, head-hunting, the other, fights between tribes of one island, which has nothing to do with head-hunting, but follows some offence, especially homicide or rape, committed on the person of a member of one tribe by a member of another. The special feature of this latter mode of warfare is that honour is satisfied when blood has been shed on each side, when peace is declared through an exchange of gifts. According to our ideas, the aggrieved party, viz. the tribe whose man has been killed, or whose woman has been raped, or stolen, should not be content until it has avenged the evil by killing or maiming one or more of the offending tribe, and the final gift should, by our moral standards, take the form of compensation. But these ideas appear to be wholly foreign to the people. On the contrary, it did not seem to be of importance which tribe first lost a man, the important point being that there should be a loss on each side. The most careful inquiry failed to reveal any custom by which the offending party made a recompense for its offence, and the concluding transaction was an exchange closely resembling that of trade. Similar customs are found in other examples of Melanesian warfare, and stress is frequently laid on the necessity for equality of loss between the two sides.

In northern Africa, as in other parts of the world, the practice by which the injury of a member of one social group may be recompensed by the offender becoming a member of the injured tribe or family, suggests that there is an idea of the integrity of the group which is much more important than the emotion of revenge given by Professor Westermarck as a cause of warfare,[1] while the Melanesian practices suggest that this concept of the integrity of the group may be closely linked with the sentiments which determine the ceremonies of " trade " exchange.

A third social institution which raises the possibility of the existence of sentiments widely different from our own is slavery. In many places, and especially in Africa, those called slaves may be captives who are utilized as a means of getting work done which would otherwise have to be performed by members of the community, while in other cases, the slaves, or rather pawns, are persons who are repaying either their own

---

[1] See p. 8.

debts or the debts of their relatives by means of their labour.

Close examination of the social functions of these so-called slaves reveals a state of affairs very different from what we ordinarily understand by slavery. Thus, there are persons in the head-hunting districts of Melanesia who are habitually called slaves by writers, when a close study of the culture shows not only the existence of sentiments towards them very different from those we associate with slavery, but also that the so-called slaves may have social functions of a very important kind. The individuals in question are captives, taken in the course of head-hunting expeditions, and they are often spoken of as " heads." Thus, one is told that the booty of an expedition amounted to fifty heads, but on further inquiry one learns that ten or twenty of these so-called heads were living persons brought home at the same time as the heads needed to satisfy immediate ceremonial needs. Further, one discovers the appropriateness of the term when one learns that these persons will provide' the heads needed on future occasions. Meanwhile their captors treat them as their own children ; they marry the women of their captors and have certain important religious functions, especially the performance of acts so sacred as to carry with them the element of danger which among such peoples is never far removed from sanctity. Moreover, I was told in the island of Vella Lavella that such a slave or head might become a chief, and that there had been recent cases of this elevation of a so-called slave to chiefly rank. It is possible that a more exact inquiry into the social status of these so-called slaves in other parts of the world would reveal similar features, or would at least show the necessity of questioning the direct application of one of our own concepts to other societies which practise slavery.

The three examples of trade, warfare, and slavery which

I have briefly considered, all betray the prevalence and importance of non-utilitarian motives in the social practices of certain peoples.

They furnish good examples of the close interdependence of different aspects of human culture which among ourselves have become so specialized that it is possible to treat them independently, and as distinct from one another, though it is probable that this independence is far from being so definite as is often supposed. A still greater interest attaching to them is that they suggest the existence of sentiments of a special kind, differing, perhaps greatly, from any prevalent in our own society. It is even possible to see in some of these a group-sentiment of a kind which we cannot easily detect among ourselves as well as a concept closely connected with and yet different from our notions of property.

II

THE CONTACT OF PEOPLES

ONE consequence of the preoccupation of ethnologists with the idea of the independent origin of custom and belief has been the neglect of the study of the principles underlying the contact of peoples, and the interaction of their cultures. In recent years we have had studies, as in the work of Huntington,[1] of the causes of migration, of the factors which have set peoples in motion, and thus acted as the starting-point of the blending of cultures. We have also had accounts, as in a recent book by Haddon,[2] of the migrations of which we have evidence in history, tradition or culture. I do not know, however, of any work which deals with the conditions which determine the results of these movements.

If we are to adopt as the main working hypothesis of ethnology that the examples of human culture now found about the earth are the complex results of the blending of peoples, and if its primary task be the analysis of this complexity, it becomes a matter of urgent necessity to understand the nature of the process of blending. We have to study how far the compound which emerges from the process is determined by the physical conditions of the country in which the blending takes place; and how far the character of the process is determined by the relative numbers, degree of culture, and other conditions, of the people who come into contact with one another.

---

[1] *The Pulse of Asia*, London, 1907.
[2] *The Wanderings of Peoples*, Cambridge, 1911.

It would be hopeless to attempt here to deal comprehensively with so vast and complex a subject, and I propose to devote this necessarily inadequate essay to the formulation of one principle, and then to inquire whether this principle can help towards the solution of two of the outstanding ethnological problems of to-day.

The contact of peoples is not a process which is limited to the past, but one which is still going on before our eyes. Let us inquire whether this process of the present may suggest a principle which will guide us to a better understanding of the past. During the last two centuries there has been going on, and still is continuing, a movement of our own people to all parts of the world. A rough survey is sufficient to show that the effects of this movement have depended largely on the nature of the culture of those whom it has reached. The more developed and highly organized the culture of a country, the less is the effect upon it of our own people. In such a country as China the effect of European influence has been slow and in amount is still very slight. On social structure and language, the effect is infinitesimally small; on religion it has been little greater; and even on material culture it has been so slight that, if all Europeans were to leave China to-morrow and the country were again to be closed, it would probably be difficult for the future archæologist to discover even the material traces of their presence, except on the sites of some coastal settlements and of a few large towns.

In India again, it is doubtful whether, except in material culture, our influence has really been much greater. We have had little effect on social structure, on the caste system, on language or on religion, and it is noteworthy that the greatest effect has been in those parts of India where the indigenous culture has remained at a relatively low level. It is only in the south that the English language and the Christian religion have obtained any hold on the people.

If now we compare this influence on China and India with that which has been exerted on such lower cultures as those of America, Africa, and Oceania, the difference is very great. The English language and the Christian religion are readily adopted; even social structure does not escape, while the effect on material culture is so great that the difficulty of the archæologist of the future will not be to discover the nature of the introduced influence; his difficulty will be to find even the traces of the indigenous cultures on which this influence has been exerted.

It may have occurred to the reader that there is one country which may seem to form an exception to the generalization I am trying to establish. The influence of European civilization upon Japan would seem at first sight to form a striking exception to the rule, that the higher the culture of a people, the less is it susceptible to external influence. It must be pointed out, however, how little has been the effect of this external influence upon the more stable elements of Japanese culture, on social structure, on language and on religion, and, further, such effect as there has been is due, not to the influence of immigrants, but to a process of a quite special kind, a process which perhaps will stand out in the future as the striking historical fact of our own times, a process in which a people of high culture have recognized their inferiority in certain of the more material arts of life, and have deliberately chosen from the culture of others just those elements which they have believed to be useful. Japan is one of those exceptions which, when we study them more closely, are found to prove the rule.

A brief survey of the effect of modern European culture throughout the world thus suggests the working of a principle, that the condition which emerges from the contact of peoples depends upon the distance which separates them in the scale of culture. With the exception I have already considered, there is no reason to suppose that this modern movement differs in any essential respect from the many which have preceded it. The difference is one of degree rather than of kind. With our improved means of transport, we now do in years what once took centuries, but it is unlikely that the principle I have sought to establish for the present is a new feature in the history of mankind. I propose, therefore, to use as a guide to the past the principle that the extent of the effect of a migrating people upon those among whom they settle, is proportional to the degree of superiority of the immigrant culture, and from this it will follow that the greater the superiority of an introduced culture, the smaller need be the number of its introducers. The special theme of this paper is that few immigrants are able to exert a deep and far-reaching influence if their culture be greatly superior to that of the people among whom they settle.

We have first to inquire what is the criterion of the superiority which allows the few to exert an influence out of proportion to their number. It is clear that we have not to do with any absolute standard of the higher or lower. The influence of an introduced culture is not determined by any absolute superiority, but by its effects on those to whom it is presented. It is the fact that an introduced culture seems to those who adopt it to be higher than their own which determines the extent of its influence. We have, then, to inquire what aspects of culture thus impress on the minds of rude peoples this notion of superiority, and here again I believe that the study of the spread of modern European influence gives us the answer. An examination of our own times makes it clear that in this direction it is material culture which counts, and counts almost alone.

High organization of social structure, a refined and exalted religion, high æsthetic ideals finding their accomplishment in works of art, a language capable of expressing the finest shades of meaning, all these are important when we have to do with settlements among those already civilized. To the uncivilized they are of small importance beside the purely material aspects of culture. It is the knife and the match, the steamship, the house and its furniture, but above all and beyond all the firearms of the European, which impress the man of rude culture and lead him to regard their possessors as beings of a higher order than himself. It is the recognition of the superiority of the material objects and arts which precedes and makes possible the acceptance of other elements of an introduced culture.[1]

An example may be given to illustrate the effect produced on a rude people by the superiority of material culture. About the year 1804, twenty-seven convicts escaped from New South Wales and found their way to the Fijian Islands.[2] The settlement of these few men had a far-reaching influence on Fiji. The supremacy of the people of Mbau and Rewa, and the manifold consequences of this supremacy were due to the help which they gave to the chiefs of those districts. This influence was due predominantly, if not entirely, to the firearms of the visitors. Owing to the effect of their weapons they were regarded as more than human, their every wish was gratified, and if they had been more worthy representatives of their race, they might have had an even greater influence. The nature of the reception of these visitors

---

[1] This statement is perhaps too sweeping. In many places we have evidence that small bodies of immigrants have been venerated because they were regarded as divine or as the ghosts of the dead, and the material culture may have formed only one factor in the production of this idea. Again, when the immigrants have been allowed to settle, any mental superiority they may have possessed cannot but have shown itself in many ways, though even here it is the manifestation of this superiority in material concerns which is most likely to impress the rude imagination.

[2] See *Fiji and the Fijians*, vol. i, by Thomas Williams, London, 1858, p. 3.

enables us to understand how great might be the influence of a body of men, no larger, but more fit to follow up the impression made by their material arts.

Further, the example shows how great an effect on culture may be produced by a body of immigrants so small as to have no appreciable effect on the physical characters of the people. Though one of the twenty-seven settlers in Fiji had no less than forty-eight children, the physical anthropologist who visits Fiji to-day would find nothing which would lead him to suspect the former presence of a body of immigrants who not long ago exerted a profound influence on the fortunes of the country.

I have now put forward as a working principle that superiority of material culture will enable a few immigrants to exert a great influence on those among whom they settle. It remains to inquire whether this principle is capable of helping towards the solution of any of the problems by which the ethnologist of to-day is confronted. For this purpose I choose two : (1) the nature of Australian culture, whether it is simple or complex, and (2) the origin of megalithic monuments, whether they belong to a single culture or have come into existence independently in different parts of the world.

The Complexity of Australian Culture

In the many works in which the Australian aborigine is held to have been the originator of human institutions, there is necessarily implied the idea that his culture is simple. If it could be shown that Australian culture is complex and contains many elements derived from without, perhaps even in ethnologically recent times, there must arise the most serious doubts whether we are justified in looking to it for material whereon to found theories of social origins. Certainly, such a procedure is wholly unjustifiable without a preliminary analysis of the complexity of its elements, and there can be little doubt that the result of this analysis would be to cut away the ground underlying many of the speculations concerning human institutions which have arisen out of the study of Australian culture.

There are few parts of the world where there seems at first sight to be so much to support the idea of unity of culture. Rarely do we find so high a degree of uniformity of physical type over a large area; rarely such similarity of custom and of institution and apparently of the underlying ideas and beliefs. The differences, and highly significant differences, are there ready to be seen by those who look for them, but it is not unnatural that under the influence of the dominant idea of the unity of this culture, they have been overlooked, and that there are ethnologists prepared to acknowledge the complexity of human culture in general, who still hold firmly to the unity of that of the Australian aborigine.

Elsewhere I have pointed to features of Australian culture which suggest its complex character.[1] The combination of two forms of social organization which elsewhere are found apart and the nature of Australian mythology seem to indicate complexity and I propose now to support these with yet another indication. Few customs of mankind take so firm a hold of his imagination as his modes of disposing of the bodies of the dead. If, therefore, Australian culture has been isolated, and is the outcome of spontaneous growth through immense stretches of time, we should expect to find much uniformity in the disposal of the dead. It is difficult to see in the environment of the Australian anything which could have led him, unaided and untaught, to evolve a variety of funeral rites.

[1] Address, Section H, British Association, 1911; *Report*, p. 490, or *Nature*, 1911, lxxxvii, 356, and *Folk-Lore*, 1912, xxiii, 307. See also pp. 158-166 of this volume.

Yet, as I have already pointed out (pp. 163-4), nearly every one of the chief known methods of disposal of the dead is practised in Australia. We find inhumation in the extended and the contracted positions; we find preservation on platforms, on trees and in caverns. There is embalming though of a simple kind, and, lastly, there is cremation.

On the assumption of the unity of Australian culture, we have to suppose that this lowly people with their relative uniformity of social structure, of art and of material culture, has yet independently evolved the chief methods of disposing of the bodies of the dead which are found throughout the world. We know the Australians to be a people of far greater mental power and initiative than the extreme simplicity and crudeness of their material culture would suggest, but it is straining the doctrine of the independent origin of human custom to the breaking-point to suppose that these people have been capable of such extensive and revolutionary changes in a department of culture where all the emotions and sentiments which influence mankind most deeply might be expected to have preserved unity and conformity to established custom.

My comparison (see p. 165) of Australian modes of disposal of the dead with those of neighbouring Oceanic peoples makes it still more difficult to accept the independent origin of the Australian practices. In this comparison, we find not merely general resemblances, but those in detail which are still more useful indications of a common source. If it should be shown, as I hope will be the case, that the Melanesian and Polynesian modes of disposal of the dead belong to the cultures of peoples who have reached these regions from elsewhere, it will, I believe, be found impossible to withhold assent to the proposition that there has been a similar introduction from without into the Australian Continent.

Further, there is an aspect of the subject about which we

can be confident. New funeral customs are not widely adopted as the result of the visits of strangers who come and go, nor can they possibly be due to visits of the Australians themselves elsewhere for trade or other purposes. People do not adopt new funeral rites merely because they see or hear of them elsewhere. If the funeral customs of Australia have been introduced from without, they have been the outcome of permanent settlements of strangers who lived and died in such close relations with those among whom they settled that the visitors were able to prescribe how their own bodies should be treated, and were so honoured, if not reverenced, that the customs they introduced have become established and time-honoured practices.

The problem before us is to reconcile this diverse influence from without with the relative uniformity of the physical type of the Australian people. I suggested on p. 162 that the solution of this problem is to be found in the introduction of the diverse funeral rites of Australia by relatively small bodies of immigrants who had so great an influence only through their possession of cultures which seemed to those among whom they settled to be vastly superior to their own.

The area of the Australian continent is so large and the natural means of travel so scanty that if the introduced cultures were brought only by small bodies of immigrants, it is unlikely that these would themselves have been able to pass to the interior in any number. The introduced elements of culture would have been carried chiefly by means of secondary movements of the earlier inhabitants who had been influenced, and thus the relative uniformity of the physical features of the Australian would become natural.

There remains to inquire what may have been the source of the superiority which, on this hypothesis, the Australians ascribed to each successive body of immigrants. We seem driven to suppose that, after each new arrival, the people reached a state in which they were once more ready to be impressed by the superiority of an external culture.

In turning to this inquiry, we come at once upon a position which seems at first sight to contradict the conclusion formulated in the preliminary portion of this essay. If it is material culture which so especially impresses rude peoples and allows small bodies of immigrants to exert so great an influence, should we not expect to find in Australia some indications of the material arts which, on my hypothesis, gave their potency to the invading cultures? We have to explain why the material culture of Australia should be so simple, why there should be such an absence of the complexity which is suggested by the ritual of death.

I have supposed that the introducers of the diverse funeral rites of Australia were but divergent streams of people who introduced similar rites into Melanesia and Polynesia. In these latter regions, we have abundant evidence of the persistence of the material arts introduced by the immigrants. On the hypothesis I have put forward, we have to suppose that these arts have disappeared in Australia.

I have dealt elsewhere with the subject of the disappearance of material arts.[1] I have sought to show that even the most useful arts may disappear among those of lowly culture, and it is essential to the argument I am now developing that this disappearance of useful arts should have taken place in Australia, and on a scale perhaps unrivalled anywhere else in the world.

On the principle I put forward, the history of Australian society presents itself as that of an isolated people dwelling in an environment which offered little inducement for the maintenance, much less for the development, of any but the simplest arts of life. Among this people I suppose that there have come at intervals bodies of immigrants, whose numbers

[1] See p. 190.

were small, but whose culture seemed so wonderful to the lowly people among whom they settled that they were able to exert a great and far-reaching influence, an influence not limited to the parts where the visitors themselves settled, but one which was carried by secondary movements throughout the length and breadth of the Australian continent.

After each new arrival and sowing of external influence, I suggest that the material culture of the visitors degenerated and had little permanent effect. It is in religious and magical rites, in myth and tradition, that the traces of these successive influences are to be sought. Owing, partly to the failure of the immigrants to implant the material arts which had been the chief cause of their influence, partly to the loss and degeneration in course of time of such arts as had made a footing in the new home, I suppose that Australian culture sank after each immigration nearly or wholly to its former level, so that each stream of external influence found a people ready to be impressed anew. The degeneration and loss of the material arts introduced from without make it possible to understand the existence of a complexity which would seem at first sight to be inconsistent with the physical uniformity of the race and with the simplicity of its material arts.

The clue to the contradiction which seems to be present in Australian culture, in its combination of evidence for simplicity and complexity, is, I believe, to be found in the principle I have put forward. It has arisen through the preponderating influence which falls to the lot of small bodies of immigrants whose culture seems great and wonderful to those among whom they settle.

Further, it seems possible that the process I have suggested may enable us to understand another peculiar feature of Australian culture. If I were asked to pick out any one character which gives the Australians so exceptional and interesting a position among the peoples of the world,

I should point to the combination of their highly complex social and magico-religious institutions, with the extraordinary crudeness of their material and æsthetic arts. I do not think that I need point out at length how naturally this would follow from the loss of useful arts which I have supposed to have taken place. A process which I have so far used only in a subsidiary hypothesis to support my main position, enables us to understand another puzzling feature of Australian culture. Not only is the incoming of small bodies of immigrants, who lose their material arts, able to explain the combination of physical uniformity with cultural diversity ; it also enables us to understand the combination of extreme material simplicity with the high degree of complexity which is shown by the social and magico-religious institutions of Australia.

Megalithic Monuments

I have next to consider whether the principle I have formulated may not help towards the solution of another problem which is now very prominently before the archæologist and the ethnologist. The monuments constructed of large rough stones found in many parts of the world have such striking similarities that to the untutored intelligence they naturally suggest a common source, and this mode of origin has also been held by many of those archæologists who have paid especial attention to the matter. Ethnologists, however, have been so under the sway of the idea that such similarities are indications of psychological, rather than of historical unity, that they have almost unanimously, at any rate in this country, rejected the possibility of the spread of the monuments from a common source. Forty years ago, a large mass of evidence pointing to historical unity was collected by Fergusson,[1] but even so recently as 1911 at the Portsmouth meeting of the British Association one of our

[1] *Rude Stone Monuments*, London, 1872.

leading anthropologists cited Fergusson's view as an example of the fate which every theory must expect which ventures to refer huma:: institutions to a common source. Before the Portsmouth meeting, however, had run its course, it seemed that the idea of cultural unity was scotched, not killed, for Elliot Smith appeared as the defender of the view that the megalithic monuments of the world are the work of people actuated by an idea which did not arise independently in many different places, but had spread from one centre.[1] He has since developed this view more fully,[2] and megalithic monuments were the subject of a discussion in 1912 at Dundee where, however, it may be noted that the weight of expert opinion was thrown almost entirely into the scale against the cultural unity of the monuments.

I need hardly say that I do not propose to attempt to deal fully with this subject. I can consider only whether we are at all helped towards the solution of this problem if we suppose that small bodies of immigrants succeeded through the superiority of their culture in introducing the practice of building these monuments.

I will consider first whether this will help us in a point which divides the advocates of cultural unity. Most of those who accept this unity suppose, as does Elliot Smith, that the idea of building the megalithic monuments, and the knowledge necessary to put this idea into execution, were not carried by one racial movement, but passed from people to people, the movement being one of culture rather than of race. So far as I know, Macmillan Brown [3] and Peet,[4] are the only open adherents of the view that the megalithic monuments of the world are the work of one people. I believe that the usual ground for the rejection of this view

[1] See *Man*, 1911, p. 176.
[2] *The Ancient Egyptians*, London and New York, 1911; *Man*, 1912, p. 173; see also pp. 168-9 of the present volume.
[3] *Maori and Polynesian*, London, 1907.
[4] *Man*, 1912, p. 174; and *Rough Stone Monuments*, London and New York, 1912.

is the physical diversity of the people who inhabit the countries where megalithic monuments are found.[1]

To most people, I find that it seems almost too grotesque for serious consideration, to suppose that there can be anything in common to the cultures of Spain and Japan, of Ireland and Madras. This dissimilarity of physical character, however, ceases to be a difficulty if the megalithic culture has been carried, not by vast movements of a conquering people, but by the migrations of relatively small bodies of men. If there once travelled widely over the world a people imbued with the idea of commemorating their dead by means of great monuments of stone, and if these people possessed a culture which seemed to those among whom they settled to be greatly superior to their own, it will follow on the principle I have put forward, that their number may have been so small as to have exerted little, if any, influence upon the physical type of those among whom they settled.

Having now considered the bearing of our principle on the dispute between the advocates of racial or cultural movement, I can turn to the main problem. I have supposed that it is superiority of culture which gives their influence to small bands of immigrants. If the carriers of the megalithic culture made their way, not by force of numbers, but by the superiority of their endowment, we have to seek for the grounds of this superiority.

It might be thought sufficient to point to the monuments

---

[1] The most cogent objection to the existence of a " megalithic race " is not to be found in the present dissimilarity of physical character or of general culture in the places where the monuments are now found, but in the long intervals which elapsed between the appearance of these monuments in different places. If archæologists are right in supposing that the megalithic monuments of Ireland were built a thousand years after those of the Mediterranean and those of Japan still another thousand years later, there can be no question of uniformity of race. No people settled on the way to these extremities of the megalithic distribution could have preserved their racial purity. Such long intervals make possible some community of racial character among the carriers of the megalithic culture, but they exclude the idea that they can have been of one race.

themselves. Such examples of human workmanship cannot but have been associated with other cultural features calculated to impress any people, much more such as we must suppose those to be among whom 'the migrants settled. I propose, however, not to be content with this easy answer, but to inquire whether we cannot define the main cause of their superiority more closely.

It is an essential feature of the scheme put forward by Elliot Smith, that the spread of the megalithic culture was closely associated with the knowledge of metals. If, as he supposes, the idea of commemorating the dead by means of large monuments of stone travelled in close company with the first knowledge of metals, we go no further in our search for the main cause which enabled the few to implant their culture. If Elliot Smith is right, metals stood in the place of the fire-arms of to-day, as the essential element of culture which allowed the few to prevail.

There is, however, a serious objection to the view that the megalithic culture had, as one of its elements, the use of metals. In many places where megalithic monuments are found, there is no evidence of their association with metals, and even where metals were present, the stone was not worked by means of them. If, as Elliot Smith supposes, megalithic monuments first arose, and only became practicable through the use of metals, the child appears to have outrun its parent in its journey through the world. We have to explain the lagging behind of the use of metal, through which the execution of megalithic monuments first became possible.

I venture to suggest that the clue to the difficulty is again to be found in the carrying of the megalithic idea by small bodies of migrating people. There is a great difference between the introduction of metals and the introduction of the art of working metals. In many parts of the world where metals are now in daily use, isolation would soon reduce

the people once more to the use of stone or shell. Small
bodies of migrating peoples would soon exhaust such metal
tools as they could take with them. Unless they discovered
metallic ores in their new home, and were able to command
the means of extracting them from the metal they needed,
they would soon be compelled to be content with the tools
of those among whom they had settled. The loss of the art
of working metal, which might seem almost inconceivable if
carried by invading hordes, spreading over large tracts of
country, becomes more easy to understand if the art belonged
to a few migrants settling among a rude people, destitute of
all but the simplest arts of life. The carrying of the megalithic culture by the few makes possible the loss of useful arts
which otherwise it would be difficult to understand.

On this assumption, it becomes possible that in some
cases the use of metals may have been lost on the way to
the extremities of the distribution of megalithic monuments.
In some of the outlying countries reached by the megalithic
culture, the migrants may already have lost the knowledge
of metal, and in these places their superiority of culture
would have been due, not to the possession of metals themselves, but to features of culture which had become possible
through the use of metal by their ancestors.

The principle which I have supposed to govern the
contact of peoples, not only removes certain difficulties which
stand in the way of the unity of the megalithic culture; it
also enables us to understand certain characteristic features
of the distribution and mode of transport of this culture.
A striking feature of the distribution of megalithic monuments
is its limitation to islands and regions of continents border-
ing on the sea. This limitation can only be accounted for
by one mode of transport. Whether the culture were carried
by one race or passed from people to people, we can be
confident that its chief, if not its only, route was on the sea.

Transmission by a seafaring people will explain the presence of the monuments on islands and in the neighbourhood of coasts, but, standing alone, it fails to explain the limitation to these situations ; there have to be explained such striking features of distribution as the total absence of megalithic monuments from the central parts of Europe and Asia. If the idea of commemorating the dead by monuments of stone had been carried through the world by conquering hordes of migrating people, this limitation of distribution would be a matter difficult to understand. The limitation to islands and coastlines suggests rather small trickling movements of a stream of people who made their way not by force of numbers or of arms, but by such superiority of material and mental endowment as made it possible for the few to implant their culture. Not only does the carrying of the megalithic culture by small bodies of people remove certain difficulties of the main problem ; it also enables us to understand one of the most characteristic features of the distribution of the monuments, the failure of their builders to construct them at any great distance from the sea.

It may be conjectured that there is reason to associate the megalithic monuments with war. The nature of many of the megalithic remains suggest that they mark the sites of great battles. Even if this were established, however, it would involve no contradiction. The example I have given from Fiji is sufficient to show how visitors peacefully received may become the instrument of success in war. We have only to suppose that the cultural development started by the strangers sooner or later took a warlike turn. The limitation of megalithic monuments to the neighbourhood of the sea suggests, however, that wars thus started did not cover a wide field. They must have failed to carry the practice of constructing monuments far from the sea, even if they succeeded in implanting other elements of culture brought by the visitors.

Further, if the megalithic culture were sea-borne, it becomes natural, if not necessary, that they should have been carried by the few. The vessels in which there journeyed the bearers of the megalithic culture must have been seaworthy and roomy craft, but it is unlikely that they could have carried large bodies of men past the open and hidden dangers of the sea, even within regions where every one acknowledges transmission. And if we accept the unity of the culture, of a culture which travelled from its birthplace to Ireland and Scandinavia, in one direction, and to Japan and the Pacific Islands in another, it is hardly possible that it can have been carried by large masses of people. We are thus led to the same conclusion as that suggested by the principle I have put forward. Both lines of argument converge, and bring us to the conclusion that, if the megalithic culture be one, it was carried by small bodies of people.

One more suggestion. May there not be a relation between the passage of the megalithic culture by sea, and its association with the use of metals ? May it not have been the knowledge of metals which first made possible the building of craft fit to carry men to such distant parts of the globe ? We know that vessels capable of long ocean voyages can be constructed without the use of metal, but if the megalithic idea had its birth in the knowledge of metals, and was fostered by their use, a great impetus must have been given to the manufacture of vessels which would make possible the dissemination of the idea throughout the world.

I believe that it will become far easier to accept the ethnological unity of the megalithic culture if we assume that it was carried by small bodies of migrating people peacefully received. The peculiar features of the distribution of the monuments, the transport of the culture by the sea, the slowness with which it travelled, all become natural if those who carried the culture were small adventurous bodies of seafarers who through the knowledge of metals had, directly or indirectly, reached a level of culture so high that they became the chiefs, perhaps even in some cases the gods, of those among whom they settled.

It is evident that the principle I put forward will become the more important the nearer we approach the extremities of the distribution of megalithic monuments. In the immediate neighbourhood of the birthplace of the megalithic idea, we should expect to find it carried by larger masses of people who may in some cases have made their way far inland. Thus, the wide distribution of the monuments in France and their extension from the Mediterranean to Brittany show movements on a scale which suggest that we are not far from the original home of the culture. It is rather in India, Japan, the Pacific Islands and South America that the problem becomes simplified by the adoption of my principle.

I began this essay with the formulation of the principle that the extent of the influence of one people upon another depends on the difference in the level of their cultures. I have now tested the value of this principle by applying it to the study of two problems which furnish prominent examples of difference of standpoint in the ethnology of to-day. In the case of Australia, my task was to reconcile cultural diversity as shown by funeral rites with physical unity. In the megalithic problem the task was rather to reconcile cultural unity with physical conditions of the utmost diversity. The application of the principle has made it possible to understand much that, without it, would be obscure and contradictory. I believe that we shall have taken a distinct step towards the solution of these problems if we assume that in each case small bodies of migrating people produced deep and far-reaching changes through the possession of a culture which seemed great and wonderful to those among whom the migrants settled.

INDEX

Printed and bound by CPI Group (UK) Ltd, Croydon, CR0 4YY

01/11/2024

01782635-0005